DIAGNOSING FOLKLORE

DIAGNOSING FOLKLORE

Perspectives on Disability, Health, and Trauma

Edited by Trevor J. Blank and Andrea Kitta

University Press of Mississippi / Jackson

www.upress.state.ms.us

The University Press of Mississippi is a member
of the Association of American University Presses.

First printing 2015

∞

Library of Congress Cataloging-in-Publication Data

Diagnosing folklore : perspectives on disability, health, and trauma /
edited by Trevor J. Blank and Andrea Kitta.

    pages cm
  Includes bibliographical references and index.
  ISBN 978-1-4968-0425-9 (hardback) — ISBN 978-1-4968-0426-6
(ebook) 1. Disabilities—Social aspects. 2. People with disabilities—
Social conditions. 3. People with mental disabilities—Social conditions. 4. Stigma (Social psychology) 5. Folklore—Social aspects.
6. Sociology of disability. 7. Disability studies. I. Blank, Trevor J.,
editor. II. Kitta, Andrea, 1977– editor.
  HV1568.D526 2015

    362.4—dc23   2015015800

British Library Cataloging-in-Publication Data available

To Erika Brady

CONTENTS

Part Three
The Performance of Mental Illness, Stigma, and Trauma

ACKNOWLEDGMENTS

This book began as a series of conversations during the annual meeting of the American Folklore Society in 2012; expanded into extended deliberations via email and social media throughout spring 2013; and by summer of that year, culminated in a call for papers that brought this volume's slate of contributors together. It has been a humbling and gratifying experience to work with such a distinguished and dedicated group of scholars, and we would like to take this opportunity to express our appreciation to the individuals whose care and support made our collective efforts such an enjoyable, stimulating, and deeply fulfilling enterprise.

First and foremost, we would like to thank our families for their love and understanding as we navigated the perpetual rush of writing, editing, and occasional disregard for the human need to sleep. To our spouses, Angelina Blank and Craig Brown, in the most *Ferris Bueller*-esque way possible: you're our [respective] heroes. We are also incredibly grateful to Craig Gill and the wonderful staff at the University Press of Mississippi for their thoughtful service and unwavering enthusiasm for this book project since its inception. The annual meetings of the American Folklore Society have consistently provided an energizing, collaborative forum in which new ideas and folkloristic discourse can emerge; the research presented herein is a testament to that fact, and we are indebted to the society and its membership for supporting our efforts to test and refine the arguments that ultimately came to populate this volume.

We have been fortunate to know and work with many special people whom we are proud to count as friends. We would like to express our appreciation to Ian Brodie, Simon J. Bronner, Anthony Buccitelli, Charley Camp, Jim Donahue, Bill Ellis, Tim Evans, Spencer Green, Bethany Haeseler, Nicholas Hartmann, Stephanie Hedge, Elissa Henken, Robert Glenn Howard, Jeana Jorgensen, Merrill Kaplan, Jim Kirkland, Linda Lee, Sabina Magliocco, Derek Maus, Jodi McDavid, Charlie McNabb, Lynne S. McNeill, Jay Mechling,

Montana Miller, Linda Moerschell, Bonnie O'Connor, John E. Price, Leonard Primiano, David J. Puglia, Jared S. Rife, Jennifer Spitulnik, Steve Stanzak, Tok Thompson, Jeff Tolbert, Elizabeth Tucker, John Paul Wallis, and John Youngblood.

Last, but certainly not least, we wish to express our gratitude to Erika Brady, to whom this book is dedicated. Erika has been a friend, teacher, and mentor to both of us, and her work in folklore and medicine has inspired and informed much of this volume. It is our honor to dedicate *Diagnosing Folklore* to her.

DIAGNOSING FOLKLORE

INTRODUCTION

The Anatomy of Ethnography: Diagnosing Folkloristics and the Conceptualization of Disability

—Andrea Kitta and Trevor J. Blank

In the wake of everyday life, where individuals and communities routinely navigate the tenuous social constructions that contextually define normalcy, the byproduct of its brooding inverse—stigma—simultaneously takes shape, coloring folk perceptions of what is normal and abnormal, sane and insane. It is a collaborative effort and countereffort, etched in symbolic interaction and internalized, then reinforced, through vernacular discourse. But "normal" is challenged, perhaps most spectacularly, in notions of disability, mental illness, and trauma. Indeed, these areas present a rich convergence of meaning where the boundaries of normalcy and "otherness" may become blurred, revealing valuable insights into the underexplored dynamics of the human condition.

Diagnosing Folklore follows in a long line of folkloristic scholarship dedicated to the study of health and stigma.[1] While past scholarship has certainly covered multiple topics from concept to practice, this volume's interrogation of ethnographic practice is meant to further stimulate dialogue on theory and fieldwork methodologies in conceptualizing folkloristic approaches to the study of disability, health, and trauma. We have chosen to bring particular attention to these three areas because, while present in many enthusiastic conference papers, panels, and academic discussions over the last five years, there is a comparative absence of corresponding, published folkloristic scholarship on the intersection of disability, health, and trauma, with a few notable exceptions.[2] This volume aims to fill the existing void by not only showcasing current ideas and debates, but also by promoting the larger study of disability, health, and trauma within folkloristics and helping bridge the gaps between the folklore discipline and disability studies.

The road to understanding disability, health, and trauma is paved in subjectivity. Stigma arises at the moment of diagnosis, the very point when the condition is named and the narrative begins. Employed as a metaphor, the word *diagnosis* aptly underscores some of the methodological challenges and considerations facing ethnographers in the study of health. Ethnography is reflexive; it is personal (Behar 1996; Campbell and Lassiter 2015:1–14; Lindahl 2004:173). By extension, ethnography is also imbued with methodological expectations and moralistic ideals that mediate and sometimes complicate the process of conducting fieldwork (Fine 1993; Fine and Shulman 2009). Accordingly, researchers must conscientiously look to the moment of diagnosis—the moment they realize that they perceive something different—to contemplate their roles, influence, and obligations in order to see beyond it. Only then should they attempt to understand the complications and impact of normalcy, mindfully self-aware and empathic yet grounded and objective.

Of course, approaching the study of disability, mental illness, and trauma necessarily problematizes the role of ethnographer and folklorist. Diagnosing people—informant or otherwise—as "the folk" inherently frames them as an individual or group that needs to be rescued, saved, or given a voice, thereby assigning them the label of "other" or "not normal." While these intentions are certainly well meant, seeking to give a voice to those who do not have one, it does beg the questions: Who are we to decide who needs to be given a voice? What marks people as "other" or "not normal"? What is the role of the ethnographer/folklorist in working with these individuals and communities? These are complicated issues that require researchers to consider both intentions and methodology.

It would be difficult to argue, at first, that disability, trauma, or mental illness is often romanticized by those who study it,[3] especially when disability is studied in the context of advocacy. However, this structure occurs in redemption narratives where the disabled person serves as nothing more than a lesson to those who are "normal."[4] Instead, scholars should attempt to act as more than ventriloquists,[5] making sure that the primary purpose of their scholarship aligns with the intent of their participants. The field of folklore has been plagued with the romanticism of "the folk" (Abrahams 1993; Mullen 2000; O'Connor and Hufford 2001; Roberts 1993; Whisnat 2008), but folklorists have not always recognized their place in that romanticism. Historically, folklore scholarship has diagnosed subjects as disadvantaged "other" and the folklorist's role as savior who attempts to rescue them. Amy Shuman suggests that the "phenomenological concept of mutual understanding (especially through empathy and the erasure of stigma) continues that legacy" (2011:151). Even when operating in the best interests of participants with advocacy as the goal, folklorists can still cast these participants in the role of victim with the academic as hero. In some situations, participants are already in this role and scholars are able to continue the paternalistic process of "studying down"; in other situations, academics actually place them in a lower status role, a process Shuman refers to as "strategic romanticism" (2011:168). Folklore scholarship seeks to give those who do not have a voice a chance to represent themselves; however, this can take participants from the realm of invisibility to hypervisibility, both of which demonstrate disproportionate power relations and obscure other experiences (Goldstein and Shuman 2012:115, 121). This hypervisibility, which seemingly gives a way for voices to be heard, can conceal and propagate power relationships.[6]

Throughout this volume our contributors employ a range of terms and concepts pertaining to the study of disability, health, and trauma. While there are common threads and approaches, we nevertheless feel that it is prudent to briefly review those which are most fundamental to this volume. First, both the editors and authors have worked with the notion of the stigmatized vernacular, as defined by Goldstein and Shuman, since it expresses "not only the emic experience of stigmatization, but also the contagion of stigma—the way it spills over beyond the topic into the means of articulation" (2012:116). In other words, stigma extends beyond the topic at hand, such as trauma, mental illness, or disability, and colors all aspects of everyday life (Goldstein and Shuman 2012). Stigma, itself, is a complicated concept to define. In addition to having multiple definitions, past scholarship has theorized levels of stigma; for example, Erving Goffman (1963) focused on the discredited and the discreditable, while Gerhard Falk (2001) studied existential and achieved stigma. For the purposes of this volume, stigma is defined as any attribute that is socially discreditable. These attributes can be physical, mental, emotional, behavioral, and/or attitudinal and have been socially determined to be undesirable. We should also note that many of the contributors to this volume have deliberately avoided using gender binaries such as "he" and "she" when discussing their informants' activities. While the editors recognize that other gender-neutral terminology is sometimes used, we have chosen to use the more common they/them or the pronoun of choice for the participant.

Throughout this book, our authors demonstrate that the goal is to create equal power relationships, but they are aware that by choosing topics and participants, value is given to certain groups over others. Scholars are in a privileged position, and while folklorists, including our contributors, choose to include participants at a high level, interpretations are divided into analytic and ethnic genres and separated out into perceptions of text and context.[7] Folklorists, as culture brokers, draw attention and recognition to traditions and groups, giving them a higher value than those groups or traditions that go unacknowledged. This is similar to the way that physicians diagnose conditions as different from what is perceived to be normal; these acts can give stigma value. Even though scholars might not understand the perceived value as it is often symbolic, it is still significant because in choosing a topic, we have elected not to study other topics.

Disability studies scholar Lennard Davis suggests that a person with an impairment is turned into a "disabled" person by the gaze of the observer and that the observer themselves become disabled in their reactions to the impaired person (1995:12). By the very act of studying a group of people, the observed are cast into a category, such as "disabled," merely by noting that they are unique enough to warrant attention, which does not allow for the dynamic process of group creation and maintenance. This acknowledgment, that the marginalized group has knowledge which has been taken for granted by the ethnographer, is remarkably similar as a discourse on normalcy. While the goal of the folklorist is to make the unknown known, offer empathy, and challenge perceptions of "normal,"[8] this does not always lead to a greater understanding of the marginalized group, unmark categories, or eliminate stigma.[9] Many of the authors in this book, including the editors, struggle with this reality in their work and attempt to dismantle perceptions of competence, normalcy, and stigma.

Disability is often a perception more than it is a reality. In a society where curb cuts and access ramps are standard, the person in a wheelchair becomes less dis-abled. When individuals post videos of people hearing for the first time after a cochlear implant with a message that indicates that hearing is the norm, we, the audience, diagnose the phenomenological experience of deafness as decidedly *ab*normal and/or "undesirable." Understanding why people share these ideas of normalcy helps unpack what narratives are tellable about disability. The narrative itself can be the difference in the perception of normalcy and the perception of participants. While these observations might seem like mere anecdotes, they make up a larger narrative about what is tellable and untellable in both private and public discourses about disability, trauma, and mental illness. Persons who fall out of the category of "normal" are keenly aware of the public narrative about them (Ferrell 2012:136); however, scholars are not always aware of their own bias.

One of the primary areas of bias comes from a dependence on the medical model of disability, trauma, and mental illness. Disability scholars have taken the focus away from the medicalization of disability and impairment, focusing rather on the phenomenology of the actual lived experience.[10] The scholars in this volume attempt to do the same, recognizing the biases in their disciplines and their own biases toward (or against) the medical model. The medical voice, as the "expert" voice, is perceived as neutral, but it is not. Those in positions of power and privilege are not outside of their own culture. For example, in Andrea Kitta's (2012) work on the anti-vaccination movement, physicians reinforce their positions of power by telling their trainees legends concerning their "right" to call child protection services in the case of a refusal to vaccinate. This legend, which will not result in any action by child protection services, is purely used as a way to demonstrate the physician's perceived power over patients and indoctrinate trainees into their new privileged position (Kitta 2012:97–102). However, in spite of their "official" positions, as with any other group, there are informal aspects of medical training that contribute to their worldview. This is an interesting transition as the informal becomes official and medicalized.[11]

Disability narratives sometimes become medicalized by others, even to the point where they become represented as the beliefs of an entire group. When folklorists and ethnographers take these dynamic experiences and put them into print, these narratives stop being a process and instead can become canon. These accounts then become the only stories that represent the group; they gain an "official" status, which in its textual form, does not grow or change as the group grows and changes, leading the experiences as they are described to exist in a sort of time warp similar to what we seen in supernatural folklore.[12] This adds to both the untellability and the stigma of these narratives.[13] Making a canon of these narratives, just like diagnosing a condition, is problematic because they change so much. This does not mean that there are no true statements, but rather that the truth of these statements is under constant negotiation due to their context (Goldstein and Shuman 2012:122). This place of privilege takes the one group's folklore and makes it official.

One of the most significant problems with the study of stigma is that it tends to not take the lived experience of those affected by stigma into account and gives a voice instead to the medicalized authority and expert over lay knowledge. Stigma extends beyond the phenomenological experience and is the outcome of a process, so it is crucial to clarify stigma from stigmatizing storylines (Bock 2012:159; Goldstein and Shuman 2012:115). When the stereotypes are persistently unchallenged, the likelihood of stigma increases exponentially, forcing individuals' identities to be solely defined as exoteric categories. Perhaps one of the roles of folklorists who study disability, trauma, and mental illness is to challenge these categories and disrupt normalcy.

Folklore scholars' treatment of narrative, which is one of providing a window into the perspectives and experiences of others, has multiple complications, not the least of which is misrepresentation (both intentional and accidental), romanticism, stigma, and privilege. However, we cannot escape the need for these "chaotic" voices to be heard. As Goldstein writes:

> I believe that it is our responsibility to write in the face of injustice, remembering always that representation and power are intertwined, and that violence, trauma, and mental illness have been largely neglected in the ethnographic literature until quite recently. (2012:191)

Even with the issues inherent to advocacy, it should be something scholars at least consider in their research. Trying to avoid that advocacy becomes a part of research may actually be impossible. One role of scholars, in addition to dismantling normalcy, can be to advocate that academics change their views of these narratives to fit the research instead of asking participants to change their narratives to fit notions of a "good" story. Sometimes, when scholars say something is a "good" story, they mean that it fits the aims of the research and will fit nicely into assumptions of what is good scholarship. If scholars "hear and 'read' these stories as they come to us, even interrupted and broken by the gaps and ruptures" without asking the stories to fit research, academics will not only respect the healing process that survivors are undertaking, but will force perceptions into a new "normal" that will push the boundaries of our discipline (Lawless 2001:58). If one is to understand the folklore discipline's complex relationship with these topics, one also must be reflexive about their individual, complex relationship with disability, trauma, and mental illness. It is unlikely that anyone has remained unscathed by these topics, which means individuals have to address their own "unsafe spaces."[14] Perhaps scholars have been reluctant to work with disability because the space that they occupy is outside of the researcher's comfort zone or too close to home. Ethnography does often "break our heart" and force us out of our comfort zone (Behar 1996). Discomfort may also lie with individual ethnographers' inherent biases and misunderstandings about disability, mental illness, and trauma, or it might be in dealing with these topics, they will have to confront their own painful experiences.

Missing in this debate is the disabled person's desire to express his or her worldview. Perhaps in certain circumstances, there is no desire to express themselves to others. This may be due to several reasons, including the fatigue of explaining themselves to those deemed "normal," a belief that their narrative will not change the stigma associated with their condition, or simply the belief that since normalcy is a social construct, it is not their responsibility to explain themselves to others. As Amy Shuman points out, "our work rarely changes the conditions of stigma that produce dehumanizing difference, even if we make it more audible or more visible" (Shuman 2011:154). Elaine J. Lawless also mentions that giving the narrative back to traumatized persons and asking them to relive that trauma may not be in their best interest (2001:58). As Shuman states:

> I've entered the world of stigma; I've gone native. And I reject all efforts to recu-
> perate my subject position by offering me an illusion of tolerance. (2011:154)

The need to give a story a voice is the result of stigma; if the stigma did not exist in the first place, there would be no story and no need to represent oneself. If scholars would like to advocate on behalf of any group, perhaps the focus should not be on understanding our participants, but rather, understanding why there are emic and etic categories. Dismantling normalcy is where researchers can make the most difference.

To be sure, the effort to meaningfully document and analyze the multifaceted folklore of health (broadly construed), trauma, and disability presents a unique set of challenges for researchers who must strive to recognize the marginalized while also remaining objective and comprehensive. But the work must be done. In this book we have brought together ten articles, each embracing a range of perspectives and methodological approaches to these areas of study. From case studies examining performance and narratives forged in response to mental illness, trauma, stigma, and/or disability, to ethnographic analyses of local knowledge and folk remedies in treating debilitating ailments outside the regular supervision of "official" medical practitioners, to theoretical discussions on disability, stigma, and normativity and the ways in which individuals work to carve out their identities in everyday life, *Diagnosing Folklore* aims to promote bold new insights, arguments, and narratives that reveal a small but compelling sample of contemporary folklore.

We have chosen to partition *Diagnosing Folklore* into three sections, each bringing a critical focus to the areas of disability, health, and trauma. Part I, "Disability, Ethnography, and the Stigmatized Vernacular," sets the tone for this volume's emphasis on fieldwork methodology and practice while dutifully chronicling the stigmatized vernacular in informants' conceptualizations of normalcy, disability, in/competency, and narrative discourse. Amy Shuman starts us off with chapter 1, "Disability, Narrative Normativity, and the Stigmatized Vernacular of Communicative (in)Competence," which builds on her previous work with Diane E. Goldstein[15] and their shared contention that folklorists can make an important contribution to the study of stigma by devoting particular attention to the process of managing how *value* is assigned, claimed, and denied in social interactions rather than focusing on categories of stigmatization. Placing ethnographic practice and folkloristic theories of communicative competence in conversation with the works of disability studies, anthropology, and sociolinguistics, Shuman endeavors to demonstrate how normativity stigmatizes individuals, especially those with intellectual disabilities (ID), and underscores the need for multiple normalcies.

Folklorist William Hugh Jansen's (1959) classic work on esoteric and exoteric folklore has frequently been used to understand how groups identify themselves and others, but this classification becomes complicated when working with individuals with intellectual disabilities who may or may not self-identify as "disabled" or understand disability as something that applies to them because it hinges on relational conceptions of normalcy. In chapter 2, "Exploring Esoteric and Exoteric Definitions of Disability: Inclusion, Segregation, and Kinship in a Special Olympics Group," Olivia Caldeira revisits Jansen's concept of esoteric/ emic and exoteric/ etic and expands on Shuman's preceding discussion of stigma and individuals with intellectual disabilities. Drawing from fieldwork with a group of Special Olympics athletes, Caldeira applies Richard Bauman's (1971) concept of differential identity to emphasize how disability is commonly used to describe others but not oneself. In doing so, she investigates new ways of understanding the concept of disability as a fluid term that is more about understanding deviance than static notions of normalcy.

In chapter 3, "Invoking the Relative: A New Perspective on Family Lore in Stigmatized Communities," Sheila Bock and Kate Parker Horigan further extend this volume's section on disability, ethnography, and the stigmatized vernacular into the narrative and familial realms. While family stories always signify the values and identities of particular groups, they also open up opportunities for individuals to contest articulations of morality and blame in contexts of stigma. Accordingly, Bock and Horigan approach the concept of family not only as a classification of a particular folk group or a descriptor of narratives' thematic content, but as a rhetorical strategy employed by narrators in contexts wherein their reputations and identities are threatened. Bringing together fieldwork materials from two independent studies—one examining accounts of personal and community experiences with Type 2 diabetes and another examining personal narratives of Hurricane Katrina survivors—the authors highlight how the concept of family serves as a rich rhetorical resource in individual accounts of community trauma by indexing material and symbolic relationships across both time and space.

Part II, "Folk Knowledge, Belief, and Treatment in Regional and Ethnic Health Praxis," shifts our attention toward the tension between lay and official understandings of disease; explanatory models of illness; and the centrality of belief in folkloristic understandings of health, wellness, and vernacular medicine.[16] Local knowledge and folk customs, in particular, play a significant role in shaping communal dietary practices and approaches to treating ailments and disease, sometimes in defiance of "official" medical knowledge and direction. In chapter 4, "Latino/a Local Knowledge about Diabetes: Emotional Triggers, Plant Treatments, and Food Symbolism," Michael Owen Jones explores several areas of Latino/a local knowledge and belief about diabetes collected around Los Angeles, California. Here again, informant narratives powerfully reflect the critical intersection of folk culture and institutional authority. Charting explanatory models regarding causes and the course of illness or disease, the folk use of plants and botanicals to lower blood glucose levels, awareness of non-nutritional meanings and uses of food—rituals, symbols, and sources of identity—regularly ignored by dieticians, self-reported "barriers" to maintaining a recommended dietary regimen, and perceptions of the social and psychological dimensions of illness that all too rarely are considered by medical personnel, Jones sheds light into how clinical and public health officials must develop culturally sensitive treatment plans that more accurately recognize and respond to local exigencies and the preponderance of emotional and environmental stress in treating diabetes within Latino/a communities.

Whether it is Los Angeles or half a world away, folk knowledge and beliefs about health and medicine carry significant weight. In chapter 5, "Interpreting and Treating Autism in Javanese Indonesia: Listening to Folk Perspectives on Developmental Difference and Inclusion," Annie Tucker shifts our discussion focus from diabetes to autism spectrum disorder (ASD). Following a year and a half of ethnographic fieldwork in Yogyakarta and Jakarta, Indonesia, Tucker observes that while the concept of autism remains comparatively new to the region, there are, in fact, operant models of developmental difference in Javanese Indonesia and a robust repertory of available responses to ASD. While weighing the benefits and challenges of adopting and mobilizing a globalized paradigm of developmental difference, Tucker illustrates how looking at meaningful embodied folk practices of inclusion might identify potentially powerful local interventions that could be disseminated, specifically describing the work of a Yogyakarta gamelan group that uses traditional music toward individually and socially therapeutic ends.

Any discussion of folklore, health, and belief should at some point turn attention toward folk healing. Part II of *Diagnosing Folklore* fittingly closes with chapter 6, "'Heal Thyself': Holistic Women Healers in Middle America," in which Elaine J. Lawless profiles a local "healing community" of women in or near Columbia, Missouri, who regularly meet and share knowledge about and practice together various healing modalities. In addition to learning from each other, she notes, the women in the group also learn new healing practices offered by healers who were visiting from other areas, so mouth-to-mouth and hand-to-hand learning take place all the time. They all claim a holistic approach, which guides their daily lives as well as their healing practices and includes attention to complex understandings of how mind, body, and spirit work in conjunction within the human body. Through the stories of these women, Lawless offers a unique glimpse into their shared corpus of knowledge and the traditional healing beliefs and practices they espouse, as well as her own place within the healing community.

Part III, "The Performance of Mental Illness, Stigma, and Trauma," brings our volume's focus back to narrative and performance in processing trauma or coping with the constraints of stigma and the need for multiple normalcies. In chapter 7, "Deranged Psychopaths and Victims Who Go Insane: Visibility and Invisibility in the Depiction of Mental Health and Illness in Contemporary Legend," Diane E. Goldstein analyzes the portrayal of mental illness in contemporary legends, focusing on the values inherent in depictions of demented killers, quietly "mad" neighbors, and psychologically damaged victims. Taken as a group and read as parallel texts, Goldstein argues that these narratives construct and present a complex of images of mental health and illness set in changing historical and cultural contexts. Together, she asserts, the narratives create explanatory categories for mental illness and convey popular understandings of "madness"; they equate insanity with visibility of difference; they explore the gendered associations of male aggression and female passivity; and they pinpoint areas of socially tolerable and intolerable deviance.

The Internet continues to serve as a dynamic locus for vernacular expression,[17] and just like their face-to-face brethren, issues of health, stigma, trauma, and disability are bound to also find vibrant refuge in the ever-present glow and availability of technologically mediated communication. YouTube, the free Internet video-sharing platform, is home to an active community of people who performatively share personal experience narratives about mental illness. Many individuals in this group heed YouTube's early call to "Broadcast Yourself" in order to publicly "put a face" to mental illness, particularly in the form of vlogs that document and share their experience.[18] In chapter 8, "Broadcasting the Stigmatized Self: Positioning Functions of You-Tube Vlogs on Bipolar Disorder," Darcy Holtgrave engages this phenomenon through a selection of vloggers who discuss bipolar disorder and the folk groups surrounding them. The parameters of YouTube inherently define and influence users' exchanges, which are mediated by digital devices and take the form of videos, video responses, text responses, the prefabricated categories of likes and views, and/or interaction with other forms of social media. Using narrative theory, Holtgrave analyzes the strategies that speakers use to negotiate their place in relation to their audience as well as their mental illness.

In chapter 9, "Tales from the Operating Theater: Medical Fetishism and the Taboo Performative Power of Erotic Medical Play," London Brickley invites readers into a fetishist community revolving around medical practices and disability where participating individuals are acutely aware of the stigmas, boundaries, and taboos of the physically disabled and mentally ill. With special consideration placed upon the relationship between the subset of individuals who have experienced disability (and/or those that yearn to), with the nuances of their physical and erotic conditions, Brickley demonstrates that fetishes are not simply deviated sexual practices, but complex constructs of identity and chosen experience. By drawing attention to perceptions of what is sexually attractive, she also points out the bias that the disabled body is unattractive, demonstrating that this ability to either see beyond the disability or find it arousing is the primary reason for the label of deviant sexual behavior.

Unfortunately, coming to terms with disability and trauma are all too familiar foes for American combat veterans, many of whom receive inadequate, delayed, or nonexistent treatment options upon returning home. We conclude Part III (and this volume, for that matter) with chapter 10, "Falling Out of Performance: Pragmatic Breakdown in Veterans' Storytelling," in which Kristiana Willsey provides new insights into the ways in which US military veterans of Iraq and Afghanistan make meaning and process trauma through the sharing of narratives. She argues that naturalizing the labor of narrative—by assuming stories are inherently transformative, redemptive, or unifying—obscures the responsibilities of the audience as co-authors, putting the burden on veterans to both share their experiences of war and simultaneously scaffold those experiences for an American public that (with the ongoing privatization of the military and the ever-shifting fronts of global warfare) is increasingly alienated from its military. Importantly, Willsey asserts that the public exhortations in which veterans tell their stories in an effort to cultivate a kind of cultural catharsis can put them in an impossible position: urged to tell their war stories; necessitating the careful management of those stories for audiences uniquely historically disassociated from their wars; and then conflating the visible management of those stories with the "spoiled identity" of post-traumatic stress disorder (PTSD).

Despite the collective breadth and independent value of these ten chapters, this volume is not intended to be an exhaustive survey of an exceedingly complex area of folkloristic inquiry. Even within the pages of this very book, contributors do not always agree with one another, nor is there a unifying theoretical or methodological orientation employed by all authors. More work is needed, but in the interim, *Diagnosing Folklore* strives to provide a new window into the contemporary dynamics and debates that surround the folkloristic study of health, trauma, disability, stigma, and everything in between. It is our sincere hope that this volume will serve as a launching point for future research, spark new dialogues, and build from and contribute to the growing wealth of folkloristic literature that engages these important subjects. Above all, *Diagnosing Folklore* aspires to exhibit an inclusive forum for contemplating the sensitive, raw, and powerful processes that shape and imbue meaning in the lives of individuals and communities beleaguered by stigmatization, conflicting public perceptions, and contextual constraints.

We, in the multiple roles we play as ethnographers, folklorists, advocates, persons with disabilities, the able-bodied and otherwise, sometimes need to do nothing more than witness. Narratives of chronic illness, of suffering, of disability are a part of what we do as folklorists. This work needs our acknowledgment perhaps more than it requires our commentary or engagement. If we do feel the need to take action, perhaps that action is best suited to being an ally, someone who supports and listens but knows that they cannot possibly understand. We can do this is a multitude of ways, such as assigning our students readings on folklore, disability, trauma, mental illness, and stigma; supporting our colleagues in their presentations at academic conferences; sharing our colleagues' work through social media; and making our conferences more accessible.[19] On behalf of the contributors, it is our hope that this volume will further discussions on the intersection of folklore, disability, trauma, and mental illness. The need for scholarship in these areas is not only theoretical, but also practical. In addition to a reconsideration of how scholars perceive normalcy and privilege, we also need to create best practices and reconsider the very nature of how we conduct fieldwork. It begins with a conversation.

Notes

1. We recognize that the following is woefully brief but hope it provides an overview of the core folkloristic efforts in the areas of disability, health, trauma, and stigma that have meaningfully informed our contributors' collective efforts before the last five years: Brady

(2001); Gaudet (1990; 2004); Goldstein (2000; 2004; 2008); Hufford (1989; 1997); O'Connor (1994); Phillips (1993); Tangherlini (1998).

2. Of course, we do not wish to minimize the valuable contributions made by the sparsely appearing bodies of folkloristic research that have made their way to publication in the last five years. Perhaps most importantly, the 2012 special issue of the *Journal of Folklore Research* (*JFR*) (vol. 49, no. 2) on the stigmatized vernacular (Bock 2012; Ferrell 2012; Goldstein 2012; Goldstein and Shuman 2012; Shuman and Bohmer 2012) made a significant impact and certainly helped spark the conversations that ultimately formed the basis of *Diagnosing Folklore*. In addition to the *JFR* special issue, see Bock (2013); Briggs (2012); Kitta (2012); and Shuman (2011). See also Blank (2013a) and Miller (2012) for folkloristic engagements with trauma in humorous and performative contexts, and Schmiesing (2014) for an analysis of disability in Grimms' fairy tales.

3. Disability has been romanticized throughout history, especially with illnesses like tuberculosis, or conditions such as the notion that the blind have a sixth sense or that their other senses are heightened or that those with special needs are psychic and are able to speak to the gods or are more in tune with nature (see Eberly 2001).

4. As Shuman (2011) notes, making someone who is disabled into a source of inspiration for others takes away their ability to participate, making them into "icons of overcoming obstacles," thus denying them a narrative other than one about triumph over odds. It also takes away the daily lived experience. In the expected narratives, disabled persons overcome their hardship once, when in reality, it is something they must do every single day. So both their experience and their experience of living with a stigmatized category are denied.

5. See Goldstein (2012); Ritchie (1993); Spivak (1988).

6. See Bock (2012:171).

7. See Shuman (chapter 1) and Caldeira (chapter 2) in this book.

8. As many ethnographers have found in their work, the unsettling parts are where scholars learn the most, and these situations, perhaps, have the most effect on our communities. Ethnography is often set up with the unfamiliar becoming familiar, but that simplifies the entire process and makes it formulaic, as if the entire purpose of ethnography was to make the unknown, known. Rather, we submit that there are many purposes of ethnography and one of those purposes is exploring discomfort, especially our own.

9. See Shuman (2011:149, 154).

10. Amy Shuman suggests that we look to phenomenology as a way of understanding narratives which are chaotic, untellable, or just hard to understand as it recognizes that this knowledge is already embodied and that the experience of self infers the experience of others (2011:167). We agree with Shuman regarding the idea that we can never truly understand another's point of view; we also agree with her notions of empathy and erasing stigma as a means of attempting to understand others. The use of the term *empathetic unsettlement* (LaCapra 1999:699; see also Shuman 2011:168) is perhaps the best means of understanding this concept. In empathetic unsettlement, ethnographers realize that they cannot share the experience of another but still attempt to understand and put themselves in that position.

11. Take, for example, Elyn R. Saks's (2008) personal experiences in the British and American medical systems as she negotiated her own mental illness. Both of these medical

systems were "official," but their training and the way they treated those with mental illnesses varied significantly. While both medical systems likely could find research and studies justifying their approach, it was a matter of training and enculturation that led them to treat their patients in vastly different ways, thus making the informal medicalized.

12. See Bennett (1987:13).

13. See Goldstein (2012:192).

14. See Goldstein and Shuman (2012:123).

15. Goldstein and Shuman's (2012) essay serves as the introduction to the aforementioned special issue of the *Journal of Folklore Research* (vol. 49, no. 2), titled "The Stigmatized Vernacular."

16. Our use of the word *praxis* is meant to convey a more holistic, practice-centered interpretation of health. As Simon J. Bronner notes: "In praxis is the idea that individuals form customary modes of behavior and thought in reaction to their perceptions of life around them and in response to the social and economic organizations in which they operate. In praxis the view of the social structure and the role of history become more important than in performance" (1988:93).

17. See, for example, Blank (2012; 2013a; 2013b; 2015); Howard (2008a; 2008b); Kaplan (2013).

18. A "vlog" is shorthand for "video blog," or a digitally recorded narrative that is posted to an individual's website or (more commonly) to a larger video hosting platform, such as YouTube. Vlogs typically feature opinionated rants or discussions about a particular theme or, in the case of online communities, a given subject matter. Vloggers, then, are individuals who post original vlogs and/or reply to and commune with others by posting vlogs. For a folkloristic primer, see Buccitelli (2012).

19. The American Folklore Society, to its credit, has worked to schedule longer breaks during annual meetings, and continuing to allow people to come and go in sessions is an excellent start. Other suggestions that might increase accessibility and inclusivity at academic conferences include providing child care (or at least the opportunity to have group child care) and creating a "quiet room" to help deal with sensory overload (which could also be used for quiet meditation, breastfeeding, prayer, and yoga or other forms of moving meditation). Other potential ideas include providing handouts (possibly in large print for the visually impaired), which might help colleagues who are not native English speakers. This practice has worked well both for the Folklore Studies Association of Canada (FSAC) and the International Society for Contemporary Legend Research (ISCLR). Additionally, if paper titles do not already make it clear, offering trigger warnings of sensitive topics before the start of our presentations may help those who have experienced trauma. Many adults with disabilities already have coping mechanisms in place, but asking if there are ways that we can improve on their experience may be another way to engage our community in these discussions. These changes need not be expensive, but they could have a significant impact on engagement and attendance at our conferences. We implore our colleagues, allied scholars, and lay readers alike to raise these and other considerations in working to cultivate more welcoming and thoughtful professional environments for all.

References

Abrahams, Roger. 1993. "Phantoms of Romantic Nationalism in Folkloristics." *Journal of American Folklore* 106 (419):3–37.

Bauman, Richard. 1971. "Differential Identity and the Social Base of Folklore." *Journal of American Folklore* 84 (331):31–41.

Behar, Ruth. 1996. *The Vulnerable Observer: Anthropology That Breaks Your Heart*. Boston: Beacon Press.

Bennett, Gillian. 1987. *Traditions of Belief: Women, Folklore, and the Supernatural Today*. London: Pelican Books.

Berger, Harris M. 2008. "Phenomenology and the Ethnography of Popular Music: Ethnomusicology at the Juncture of Cultural Studies and Folklore." In *Shadows in the Field: New Perspectives for Fieldwork in Ethnomusicology*, ed. Gregory Barz and Timothy J. Cooley, 62–75. Oxford: Oxford University Press.

Blank, Trevor J. 2012. *Folk Culture in the Digital Age: The Emergent Dynamics of Human Interaction*. Logan: Utah State University Press.

———. 2013a. *The Last Laugh: Folk Humor, Celebrity Culture, and Mass-Mediated Disasters in the Digital Age*. Folklore Studies in a Multicultural World Series. Madison: University of Wisconsin Press.

———. 2013b. "Hybridizing Folk Culture: Toward a Theory of New Media and Vernacular Discourse." *Western Folklore* 72 (2):105–30.

————. 2015. "Faux Your Entertainment: Amazon.com Product Reviews as a Locus of Digital Performance." *Journal of American Folklore*, forthcoming.

Bock, Sheila. 2012. "Contextualization, Reflexivity, and the Study of Diabetes-Related Stigma." *Journal of Folklore Research* 49 (2):153–78.

————. 2013. "Staying Positive: Women's Illness Narratives and the Stigmatized Vernacular." *Health, Culture and Society* 5 (1):150–66. http://hcs.pitt.edu/ojs/index.php/hcs/article/view/125.

Brady, Erika. 2001. *Healing Logics: Culture and Medicine in Modern Health Belief Systems*. Logan: Utah State University Press.

Briggs, Charles L. 2012. "Toward a New Folkloristics of Health." *Journal of Folklore Research* 49 (3):319–45.

Bronner, Simon J. 1988. "Art, Performance, and Praxis: The Rhetoric of Contemporary Folklore Studies." *Western Folklore* 47 (2):75–101.

Buccitelli, Anthony Bak. 2012. "Performance 2.0: Observations toward a Theory of the Digital Performance of Folklore." In *Folk Culture in the Digital Age: The Emergent Dynamics of Human Interaction*, ed. Trevor J. Blank, 60–84. Logan: Utah State University Press.

Campbell, Elizabeth, and Luke Eric Lassiter. 2015. *Doing Ethnography Today: Theories, Methods, and Exercises*. Malden, MA: Wiley-Blackwell.

Davis, Lennard J. 1995. *Enforcing Normalcy: Disability, Deafness and the Body*. New York: Verso.

Dorst, John. 1989. *The Written Suburb: An American Site, An Ethnographer's Dilemma*. Philadelphia: University of Pennsylvania Press.

Eberly, Susan Schoon. 1988. "Fairies and the Folklore of Disability: Changelings, Hybrids and the Solitary Fairy." *Folklore* 99 (1):58–77.

Falk, Gerhard. 2001. *Stigma: How We Treat Outsiders*. Amherst, NY: Prometheus Books.

Ferrell, Ann. 2012. "'It's Really Hard to Tell the True Story of Tobacco': Stigma, Tellability, and Reflexive Scholarship." *Journal of Folklore Research* 49 (2):127–52.

Fine, Gary Alan. 1993. "Ten Lies of Ethnography: Moral Dilemmas of Field Research." *Journal of Contemporary Ethnography* 22 (3):267–94.

Fine, Gary Alan, and David Shulman. 2009. "Lies from the Field: Ethical Issues in Organizational Eothnography." In *Organizational Ethnography: Studying the Complexities of Everyday Life*, ed. Sierk Ybema, Dvora Yanow, Harry Weis, and Frans Kamsteeg, 177–95. Thousand Oaks, CA: SAGE Publications.

Gaudet, Marcia. 1990. "Telling it Slant: Personal Narrative, Tall Tales, and the Reality of Leprosy." *Western Folklore* 49 (2):191–207.

———. 2004. *Carville: Remembering Leprosy in America*. Jackson: University Press of Mississippi.

Goffman, Erving. 1963. *Stigma: Notes on the Management of Spoiled Identity*. Upper Saddle River, NJ: Prentice-Hall.

Goldstein, Diane E. 2000. "'When Ovaries Retire': Contrasting Women's Experiences with Feminist and Medical Models of Menopause." *Health* 4 (3):309–23.

———. 2004. *Once Upon a Virus: AIDS Legends and Vernacular Risk Perception*. Logan: Utah State University Press.

———. 2008. "Imagined Lay People and Imagined Experts: Women's Use of Health Information on the Internet." In *Global Science and Women's Health*, ed. Cindy Patton and Helen Loshny, 25–49. Youngstown, NY: Teneo Press.

———. 2012. "Rethinking Ventriloquism: Untellability, Chaotic Narratives, Social Justice, and the Choice to Speak For, About, and Without." *Journal of Folklore Research* 49 (2):179–98.

Goldstein, Diane E., and Amy Shuman. 2012. "The Stigmatized Vernacular: Where Reflexivity Meets Untellability." *Journal of Folklore Research* 49 (2):113–26.

Howard, Robert Glenn. 2008a. "Electronic Hybridity: The Persistent Processes of the Vernacular Web." *Journal of American Folklore* 121 (480):192–218.

———. 2008b. "The Vernacular Web of Participatory Media." *Critical Studies in Media Communication* 25 (5):490–513.

Hufford, David. 1989. *The Terror that Comes in the Night: An Experience-Centered Study of Supernatural Assault Traditions*. Philadelphia: University of Pennsylvania Press.

———. 1995. "The Scholarly Voice and the Personal Voice: Reflexivity in Belief Studies." *Western Folklore* 54 (1):57–76.

———. 1997. "Introduction." *Southern Folklore* 54 (2):1–14.

Jansen, William H. 1959. "The Esoteric-Exoteric Factor in Folklore." *Fabula* 2 (3):205–11.

Kaplan, Merrill. 2013. "Curation and Tradition on Web 2.0." In *Tradition in the Twenty-First Century: Locating the Role of the Past in the Present*, ed. Trevor J. Blank and Robert Glenn Howard, 123–48. Logan: Utah State University Press.

Kitta, Andrea. 2012. *Vaccinations and Public Concern in History: Legend, Rumor, and Risk Perception*. Routledge Studies in the History of Science, Technology and Medicine. New York: Routledge.

LaCapra, Dominick. 1999. "Trauma, Absence, Loss." *Critical Inquiry* 25 (4):696–727.

Lawless, Elaine J. 2001. *Women Escaping Violence: Empowerment through Narrative*. Columbia: University of Missouri Press.

Lindahl, Carl. 2004. "Afterword." *Journal of Folklore Research* 41 (2–3):173–80.

Miller, Montana. 2012. *Playing Dead: Mock Trauma and Folk Drama in Staged High School Drunk Driving Tragedies*. Logan: Utah State University Press.

Mullen, Patrick B. 2000. "Belief and the American Folk." *Journal of American Folklore* 113 (448):119–43.

O'Connor, Bonnie B. 1994. *Healing Traditions: Alternative Medicine and the Health Professions*. Philadelphia: University of Pennsylvania Press.

O'Connor, Bonnie B., and David J. Hufford. 2001. "Understanding Folk Medicine." In *Healing Logics: Culture and Medicine in Modern Health Belief Systems*, ed. Erika Brady, 13–35. Logan: Utah State University Press.

Phillips, Marilyn J. 1993. "Straight Talk from 'Crooked' Women." In *Feminist Theory and the Study of Folklore*, ed. Susan Tower Hollis, Linda Pershing, and M. Jane Young, 396–410. Urbana: University of Illinois Press.

Ritchie, Susan. 1993. "Ventriloquist Folklore: Who Speaks for Representation?" *Western Folklore* 52 (2–4):365–78.

Roberts, John. 1993. "African American Diversity and the Study of Folklore." *Western Folklore* 52 (2–4):151–71.

Saks, Elyn R. 2008. *The Center Cannot Hold: My Journey through Madness*. New York: Hyperion.

Schmiesing, Ann. 2014. *Disability, Deformity, and Disease in the Grimms' Fairy Tales*. Detroit: Wayne State University Press.

Shuman, Amy. 2011. "On the Verge: Phenomenology and Empathic Unsettlement." *Journal of American Folklore* 124 (493):147–74.

Shuman, Amy, and Carol Bohmer. 2012. "The Stigmatized Vernacular: Political Asylum and the Politics of Visibility/Recognition." *Journal of Folklore Research* 49 (2):199–226.

Spivak, Gayatri Chakravorty. 1988. "Can the Subaltern Speak?" In *Marxism and the Interpretation of Culture*, ed. Cary Nelson and Lawrence Grossberg, 271–313. Urbana: University of Illinois Press.

Tangherlini, Timothy R. 1998. *Talking Trauma*. Jackson: University Press of Mississippi.

Whisnat, David. 2008. *All That Is Native and Fine: The Politics of Culture in an American Region*. Chapel Hill: University of North Carolina Press.

PART ONE

Disability, Ethnography, and the Stigmatized Vernacular

Disability, Narrative Normativity, and the Stigmatized Vernacular of Communicative (in)Competence

—Amy Shuman

> For every society, the relation between normal and special modes of behavior is one of complementarity. That is obvious in the case of shamanism and spirit possession; but it would be no less true of modes of behavior which our own society refuses to group and legitimize as vocations. For there are individuals who, for social, historical, or physiological reasons (it does not much matter which), are sensitive to the contradictions and gaps in the social structure; and our society hands over to those individuals the task of realizing a statistical equivalent (by constituting that compliment, "abnormality," which alone can supply a definition of "the normal").
> —CLAUDE LEVI-STRAUSS (1987 [1950]:19)

As Claude Levi-Strauss argues, the normal and the "special" are not discrete categories but instead are mutually dependent, formed within particular cultures, as part of the social structures. Norms are always relative and produce exclusions and stigmatizing practices. Folklorists and anthropologists have identified the multiple normativities of disenfranchised groups. However, within the academic discourses of folklore and anthropology, normativity itself remains relatively unchallenged. In undertaking research with disenfranchised groups, folklorists often promote the positive value of disenfranchised groups, a move that I have described as the effort to recuperate our subjects of study, often as a matter of appreciation (Shuman 2007).[1] This practice is perhaps most familiar in folklore studies' legacy of romantic advocacy, a legacy that has sometimes resulted in a celebratory stance that can reinforce the marginalizing status of exotic others (Abrahams 1993; Ritchie 1993).

For the most part, this cost has not been considered detrimental, especially when the outcome has been greater visibility and sometimes access to resources for otherwise disenfranchised groups, though our efforts to assert the value of the groups we study does not necessarily change their status (Ritchie 1993). From the perspective of disability studies, the efforts toward recuperation look like nothing more than paternalism, and the celebratory turns out to be restigmatizing, reaffirming the disenfranchising systemic inequities.[2] Disability studies begins with a critique of sympathetic approaches to people with embodied experiences marked as different (Rousso 2013). As Lennard Davis writes: "Disability studies, for the most part, shuns this unequal power transaction in favor of advocacy, investigation, inquiry, archeology, genealogy, dialectic, and deconstruction. The model of a sovereign subject revealing or reveling in that subjectivity is put into question" (2006: xvii). The disciplinary imperatives to see others as they see themselves (folklore) and to critique the sympathetic and the celebratory (disability studies) are not necessarily contradictory, and this essay is one effort to explore that conversation, in particular through the lens of normativity and the intersections among narrative, folklore, the ethnography of communication, and disability studies. As a starting point for this conversation, I argue that implicit and uncritical assumptions about normativity can underlie the folklorist's efforts to see people as they see themselves and that letting people speak for themselves as an alternative to the celebratory is not as simple as it seems. Concepts of communicative competence are central to both issues.

Research on folklore and the ethnography of speaking often explicitly argues for multiple normalcies, at least insofar as each group has its own parameters for what counts as normal and narrative. Countering ethnocentrism, ethnographers generally have argued for multiple normalcies but have nonetheless maintained the implicit ideas of norms and normality, a perspective critiqued by disability studies. Narrative studies similarly depend on both what might be described as normative modes of telling a coherent story (Linde 1993) and on opportunities for counternarratives and alternative assessments of what is tellable; who can tell; and as a consequence, how normalcy is negotiated.

As a methodology, the ethnography of communication defends the idea of multiple normalcies, lending itself to a situated, localized, vernacular approach to normalcy. In our essay for the special issue of the *Journal of Folklore Research* on "The Stigmatized Vernacular," Diane Goldstein and I suggested that folklore research can make an important contribution to the study of stigma by attending not to the categories of what is stigmatized, but instead by observing this process of "managing" how value is assigned, claimed, and denied in social interactions. We deliberately chose the term *vernacular* to describe popular or folk performances because it is a term that conveys value. Although "vernacular" has been reconfigured positively, for example in the study of "vernacular architecture," it also conveys the idea of the nonstandard or low. Our discussions in *JFR*, and mine in this essay, are part of a larger conversation on folklore and value.

In this chapter, I build on folkloristic understandings of the stigmatized vernacular by additionally addressing questions of normalcy and stigma in everyday life. Erving Goffman described stigma in terms of the "management of spoiled identity." The particular area of disability I address in this essay, communicative competence/incompetence, has had a central role in folklore scholarship generally, though the concept of competence almost always refers to virtuosity in performance and does not imply incompetence as its opposite.[3] As studied through the framework of the ethnography of communication, narrative research embraces multiple normalcies, including the co-production of narrative that I will discuss here. I first review some of the potential intersections between disability and folklore studies and then turn to a close examination of communicative competence/incompetence framework as articulated by Dell Hymes in his outline of the ethnography of communication (Gumperz and Hymes 1972).

The discipline of disability studies established itself as an alternative to medicalized discourses about the body. In contrast to medicalized identities that sort people into categories based on a diagnosis, disability studies challenge authoritative structures of knowledge production and insist on knowledge production as embodied, and further, as embodied by different bodies with different means of perception producing knowledge from different bodies (Michalko in Corker and Shakespeare 2002:175; see also Docherty et al. 2005). For folklorists, this is similar to the familiar and important methodology of attempting to understand others as they understand themselves, but disability studies takes the method a step or two further by examining how authoritative claims to knowledge are implicated in conceptions of normalcy.[4] Folklorists have always been willing to recognize multiple "normals," but although both folklore and anthropology have awakened people to the idea of multiple cultural perspectives, worldviews, and so on, as the earlier quotation from Levi-Strauss indicates, often those cultures are considered to be governed by a form of normalcy. Here I ask how Dell Hymes's concept of communicative competence might be considered an example of the pervasiveness of the normal in folklore research.

Ethnographies of disability are, for the most part, studies of culture on the margins.[5] Importantly, however, and this is why ethnography is so important, the margins are not the same for every culture, and life on the margins can be described as stigma, as liminal, or as transgressive, among other possibilities. In particular, disability studies offers the possibility of understanding how life on the margins is reconfigured, a framework I'll return to in my conclusion.[6] Anthropologists and folklorists have identified the categories that govern social life for members of a group; disability studies expands that project to include identifying how those categories produce exclusions to membership and how those exclusions are central to understanding any society.

The term *normative* is used as a neutral term in folklore discussions. In *The Study of American Folklore*, in a section titled "Folk, Normative, Elite," Jan Harold Brunvand uses normative to mean "popular, mass, mainstream" (1978:8–10), and the normative is the middle "level of culture" between folk and elite. The normative in Brunvand's chart includes popular romance novels, nonprescription drugs, and tract development houses. Interestingly, then, for Brunvand, the normative is not the traditional. For other folklorists, the "normal" refers to the natural, for example, "the normal context for riddling" in Kenneth Goldstein's discussions of fieldwork in Scotland (1963:302).

In a foundational 1968 article outlining the performance approach to folklore, Roger Abrahams uncritically assumes a normative stance toward performance. Borrowing from Bascom's four functions of folklore, Abrahams states, "Folklore functions normatively, as a cohesive force" (1968:146). Bascom's oversimplified claim for the normative function of folklore remained unquestioned in the Abrahams model and indeed in much other folklore scholarship.[7]

Today, from the lens of disability studies, the word "normal" has become highly charged in ways that it wasn't when Abrahams, Kenneth Goldstein, or Brunvand used it in discussions of the category of folklore. Ethnographers and disability studies scholars Ray McDermott and Herve Varenne interrogate the concept of the normal from the perspective of multiple abilities:

> Culture, the great enabler, is disabling. *Culture* is generally taken to be a posi-
> tive term. If there is anything people do naturally, it is that they live culturally
> in groups, with goals, rules, expectations, abstractions, and untold complexities.
> For every skill that people gain, there is another that is not developed for every
> focus of attention, something is passed by; for every specialty, a corresponding
> lack ... being in a culture is a great occasion for developing abilities, or at least
> for having many people think they have abilities. ... Being in a culture is a great

occasion for developing disabilities, or at least for having many people think that they have disabilities. (1995:331–32)

As with all critical assessments of formerly unchallenged terms, the term *normal* can become taboo, creating its own enforced boundaries of political correctness and then silencing discussions of the most difficult topics. In contrast, by probing folkloristic conceptions of normal, and more particularly, communicative competence, through the lens of disability studies critiques, we can open up, rather than close down, discussion of communicative competence.

The concept of communicative competence is a cornerstone of the ethnography of communication and, by extension, of folkloristic performance analysis. Heritage and Atkinson write, "The central goal of conversation analytic research is the description and explication of the competences that ordinary speakers use and rely on in participating in intelligible, socially organized interaction" (1984:1). The implicit normalcy of ordinary speakers is assumed here, but Hymes did not presume a hegemonic mainstream. To the contrary, he proposed the concept of communicative competence as a central dimension of his investigation of language inequalities. It afforded the possibility of understanding differences within frameworks of communicative resources and repertoires rather than as deficits. This situated, contextualized understanding of communicative differences corresponds with recent discussions in disability studies, also interested in challenging deficit models (Kovarsky and Crago 1990–1991:44). However, the concept of communicative competence, part of Hymes's model for studying the ethnography of communication, explicitly and implicitly relies on normative systems, thus coming up against the disability studies' critiques of normalcy.[8]

Using an ethnography of communication framework, Val Williams similarly explores "the way ordinary resources of social interaction are used in particular contexts by and with people with intellectual disabilities" (2011:1). Instead of identifying deficits, she identifies how people manage to communicate differently and how closer attention to these differences in actual interactive, inclusive conversations reveals greater abilities than are usually assumed for individuals with intellectual disabilities, measured out of context. Building on Williams's work, I consider two examples of co-produced narrative in which individuals with communicative disabilities and their interlocutors manage to understand each other. I argue that their co-production of narrative qualifies as competent and that it provides an illustration of how we might understand multiple normalcies in narrative performance.

The first example is from a British reality television show, *The Specials*, that showcases the lives of individuals with intellectual disabilities who share a group home. Each episode depicts the daily life and activities of the participants. In one episode, Lucy has been told that she has been eating too much food at her job at a Heart Association thrift store. The careworker, who is on camera, explains this to Lucy and tells her that she is in danger of losing the job. Then, in a second scene, a different careworker, off camera, is talking to Lucy, who tells a narrative about her current problems:

The Specials Episode 8[9]

(Scene 1: Lucy and Dafydd the careworker in a doorway)
NARRATOR: Back home, Dafydd needs to speak to Lucy.
She's been eating too much at work.
DAFYDD: Three sausages, curry, packed lunch, biscuits, cakes.
They've put a padlock on the door
Because
Cake and biscuits
Have been going missing
So if you can't
You know
Do it
If you can't control your eating Lucy
You're gonna lose that job

(Scene 2): Lucy sitting on the floor next to her bed, crying
FEMALE CAREWORKER (off camera): Oh Lucy.
LUCY: At the moment
There's a lot of things going on
My family
It is different
This time
It's different
This time

CAREWORKER 2: What's different this time, darling?
LUCY: My family
The thing
The thing is
Dad has got his solicitor (subtitled)

Solicitors
And my mom as well
My Mom is complainin
About my Dad
(she points) he doesn't (want) to come back
That's what hurts mom

CAREWORKER 2: That hurts your mom?

LUCY: Yes
He doesn't want to come back
CAREWORKER 2: I'm sorry it upsets you so much

LUCY: It is

CAREWORKER 2: Do you think that's why you're eating
Because
you're comfort eating
LUCY: That's what it is
That's what it is.

In the second scene, Lucy and the careworker display mutual understanding of the topic, competent turn taking, and attention to the structure and organization of the talk in their interaction, and Lucy communicates emotion and affect. Put simply, they understand each other and also, importantly, coproduce understanding of the problem at hand: why Lucy has been eating at work. They negotiate a gap between the topic of Lucy's mother being upset and Lucy being upset.

Dafydd, another careworker, tells the initial narrative, about the padlock being placed on the door at work because "cake and biscuits have been going missing." The second scene is a response to this problem. In the second scene, Lucy and the female careworker share expectations in their recognition of Lucy's narrative as an explanation, which the careworker later re-articulates.[10]

Lucy's narrative hinges on the connection between her eating and the problems in her family. She first establishes the connection by saying, "It's a lot of things going on." Lucy and the careworker collaboratively negotiate what "it" refers to. Referring to her father, Lucy says, "He doesn't want to come back," and the careworker responds, "I'm sorry it upsets you so much." Here the careworker provides the evaluation, the fact that the problems are upsetting Lucy. Again, the careworker provides the explanation for the overeating by asking the question, "Do you think that's why you're eating. Because you're comfort eating?" Thus, the careworker helps to articulate the connection between the "it" that is upsetting Lucy so much (her family's problems, or more specifically, her father not wanting to come back) and Lucy's eating habits at work. The coherence of the narrative requires this collaborative, interactive exchange, and it's possible that Lucy would not articulate the metanarrative connection between her family distress and her eating at work more explicitly on her own. In this case, as others have pointed out more generally in conversational narrative, communicative competence depends upon the co-production of meaning (Ochs, Smith, and Taylor 1989). In her study of the discourse of careworkers and individuals with intellectual disabilities, Val Williams observes many such instances of co-produced meaning. This co-production of meaning qualifies as communicative competence generally, but in Goffman's terms, when one of the interlocutors has a communicative disability, the communication is *dis*qualified and stigmatized as not competent (Goffman 1963). The problem may be, at least in part, the way that individual telling is privileged such that co-narration is not recognized as "normal." Ochs, Smith, and Taylor point out, "Cognitive approaches tend to focus on *individual* tellings and retellings of stories without attending to the fact that stories are often if not typically collaboratively produced, that is, *co-narrated*, by those participating in the social interaction" (1989:41).

The following narrative, also an exchange between a careworker (A) and an individual with intellectual disabilities and communicative disabilities (L), provides another example of this collaborative, interactive production of narrative.

A: How about that OSU game
L: I went with my buddy Sarah
A: You WENT
L: I went with Sarah
A: Did you see the long pass to Devin Smith?
L: Braxton Miller passed to Devin Smith
A: What was the final score?
L: Ohio State have 33 Wisconsin 29
A: That game came down to the wire
L: Close game. WE WON
A: Did you go down on the field?
L: No. Mom picked us up
Sarah hugged me.

On the face of it, this conversation displays male competence in talk about sports. The eclipsed references are conventional for sports talk, in which participants not only share but also often perform a referential repertoire, resulting in an economy of discourse. Also, as in typical in sports talk, the narrative is co-produced, with in this case the careworker asking questions to which L responded. The careworker articulated the evaluation, "That game came down to the wire," repeated by L, saying "Close game" and adding, "WE WON," shouted as a performance of a response to the final moments of the game. Further, L returns to his initial topic, the fact that he went with his buddy Sarah, and for L, the important conclusion is not only the final winning score but also the concluding celebratory hug. Thus, in this narrative, L not only co-produced an acceptable narrative about the game; he also took control of the narrative.

The conversation is typical of L's communication. For example, L would typically say, "close game," rather than "It was a close game." In some situations, "close game" would be regarded as incomplete, and a speaker unable to produce a more complete sentence would be considered incompetent,[11] but in sports talk, it's unmarked. In sports talk, L is able to meet the requirements of both the referential and expressive dimensions of communicative competence (Hymes 1973:193), but in other genres, his referential and/or expressive uses might be negatively evaluated. Importantly, A and L produce a co-narrated discussion of sports. Like Lucy's careworker, A is attuned to L's communicative repertoire and abilities; however, the coherence of not only this exchange but all sports talk of this kind depends on co-narration. As Lars-Christer Hydén and Eleonor Antelius point out, co-narration is typical of many speaking situations among people both with and without communication difficulties (2011:8).

Co-narration serves multiple purposes, for example, as it is a means to collectively solve problems at the dinner table (Ochs, Smith, and Taylor 1989:241). Lucy's story works this way, with the careworker and Lucy together figuring out why she is eating too many biscuits at work. As Ochs, Smith, and Taylor point out, "co-constructed, unfolding settings orient and reorient a story throughout its telling" (244). In Lucy's story, Lucy first shifts her orientation from the padlocked cabinet to her family problems, and then the careworker reorients the narrative to articulate the connection to the family problems as an explanation for the biscuit eating. The careworker's reorientation serves as a meta-narrative link. Like Lucy, L performs a reorientation without a meta-narrative move when he ends the story with "Sarah hugged me." This phrase can be seen as a coherent response to the question about going onto the field, but it is out of order. First Sarah hugged him; then his mom picked him up. However, for L, the two phrases are both answers to the question of how he celebrated the end of the game. His mom picking him up is a practical answer. L reorients his answer to respond to the fact of the win, so he adds, "Sarah hugged me." For both Lucy and L, reorientation includes a shift in attention between frames. If we were to mark a difference in cognitive competence in these narrative productions, it would be in the fact that Lucy and L do not articulate meta-narrative frame shifts. However, the use of meta-narrative frame shifts is not a marker of greater ability, and individuals with and without intellectual disabilities produce narratives with and without meta-narration.

Both L's sports talk and Lucy's narrative satisfy Hymes's three requirements for communicative competence: verbal repertoire, language behavior, and linguistic routines (1971:58). In particular, they demonstrate competence of verbal repertoire and linguistic routines. At the same time, neither Lucy nor L would not be judged as competent speakers, mostly because of their articulation problems but also because of their reliance on their communicative partners to create a coherent narrative. Both of the careworkers may have modified their communication to match L and Lucy, and although in most conversations, this is a sign of competence, when one of the speakers has obvious articulation problems, the modification can serve as a sign of incompetence. The issue, then, is not the communication itself, but attitudes toward it. Lucy and L could be seen as competent narrators who meet the primary requirements for a coherent narrative. Assessments of them as less than competent narrators are attached to other signifiers, especially the fact that they have intellectual disabilities.

Conclusion: Reconsidering Narrative Normativity

The larger question framing questions of communicative competence is how a person's intelligibility makes him or her illegible in other categories of citizenship. We can recognize the gaps and how they are filled in a conversation, but when those gaps become signs of in/competence, rather than of mutual understanding, they are open to new significations. We can ask whether the careworkers' ability to translate, to be in a conversation with Lucy or L, depends on sympathy, on the willingness to understand across neurodiversities, or on not seeing the other as repugnant. At this point, once these signifiers take hold, instead of recognizing varieties of normal, differences become naturalized as non-normative.[12] Co-production of narrative, then, becomes naturalized as an exception, and within that exception, the co-production of narrative by a person with intellectual disabilities is stigmatized as incompetent.

Communicative competence is a deeply normative system, which, as Ochs, Smith, and Taylor (1989) point out, depends on etic systems that can keep in place labels of incompetence.[13] To push the point further, it assumes that speech itself is normative, a point challenged by theorists of deafness.[14] Narrative is additionally normative. Lars-Christer Hydén and Eleonor Antelius point out that "persons with communicative disabilities are often involved in storytelling that does not necessarily conform to the conventional expectations of what constitutes a narrative" (2011:1). In their research with individuals who have had brain injuries, they observe, "Storytellers who experience troubles in telling stories are often quite inventive in organizing the interaction in order to appear as the primary storytellers" (2011:3). Drawing on Erving Goffman's concept of the animator as someone who assists in the production of a narrative, Hydén and Antelius discuss co-narration as produced through embodiment and as part of a network of social relations. Lucy and L could be seen as similarly inventive in organizing their interactions as part of a social network.

Narrative normativity is often discussed in terms of counternarratives or subversive accounts. For example, Michael Herzfeld describes the adage "honor among thieves" as "the normativity of the subversive" (1979:72) in narratives about animal thieves in Crete. The adage provides a paradoxical rationale in defiance of societal norms. Disability studies also points to counternarrative as a cultural resource for subversion of dominant paradigms of normalcy and additionally is interested in the pervasiveness of the dominant paradigms and the use of narrative to sustain them. The examples I have discussed here are not counternarratives that might disrupt the category of normal conversation; to the contrary, my discussion of Lucy's and L's narratives asks whether the category of normal conversation might be expanded to include their co-production of narrative.

In disability studies, a primary critique of narrative normativity has focused on redemptive and inspirational narratives as supporting the dominant paradigms of ableism. (Rousso 2013). In contemporary Western culture, one of the most familiar representations of disability is a story of overcoming difficulties.[15] Writing about illness narratives, Thomas Couser writes, "The narrative formula of 'overcoming' impairment—rather than challenging disability (though the two are not always easy to distinguish)—has its drawbacks. A high-achieving with an obvious impairment is always in danger of becoming a Supercrip, an Inspirational Disabled Person who overcomes impairment through pluck and willpower" (1997:203). As disability studies

scholars have pointed out, overcoming narratives (as they are referred to frequently) perform an erasure by preferring the story of overcoming adver-
sity over any other narrative (Garland-Thomson 2005; Mitchell and Snyder
2000). Such narratives, disability studies scholars argue, make people with
disabilities even more invisible or even more stigmatized by requiring everyone to provide an inspirational narrative of overcoming their differences.
Refusing the inspirational narrative is a primary trope of disability studies
today. The disability studies' critique of overcoming, inspirational narratives
provides a framework for critiquing the imposition of the normative in any
domain (including efforts in folklore to recuperate disenfranchised subjects).
From the perspective of disability studies, any imperative narrative, whether
celebratory or tragic, imposes a script that potentially reinforces stigmatizing
attitudes and practices and potentially erases or makes invisible the subjects
represented in the narratives. Disability studies provides a powerful critique
of the dangers of normativities, even the multiple normalcies that are so
foundational in ethnographic research.

In their article on language ideologies, Judith Irvine and Susan Gal
observe that "differentiation is ideologically mediated, both by participants
and by its observers . . . linguistic differentiation is not a simple reflection of
social differentiation or vice versa" (2000:76). Their article offers a critique
of the Hymesian conception of speech communities that, "though useful for
understanding the organization of local repertoires, nevertheless neglected
larger boundary relationships, cultural oppositions, borders, and conflict"
(2000:75). Disability is a good example of a boundary relationship that
establishes exclusions based on assessments of competencies. Within speech
communities, people who speak differently can be labeled as less competent,
whether due to differences in dialect, in language acquisition level, or cognitive ability. Although disability studies research begins by observing that the
label "disabled" is ideologically motivated, the next step is to identify multiple
competencies.[16]

I have proposed co-narration in conversations including people with
intellectual disabilities as an example of multiple competencies. As a caution,
Val Williams observes that privileging the co-production of such narratives
can serve to erase any recognition of individuals speaking for themselves,
without such co-production (2011). Certainly, the independent production of
one's own narrative has been used to legitimate a particular sense of self.[17]
However, as we can see in Lucy's and L's narratives, co-narration can quite
adequately establish and negotiate a sense of self.

I have made the case that L's and Lucy's conversations do in fact manage
to satisfy the situated, cultural requirements of communicative competence,

taking account of the co-production of narrative. This assertion, however, is unlikely to be sufficient, because on the other hand, Lucy and L might nevertheless be assessed as incompetent, whether because they depend on co-narration or because they do not provide the meta-narrative shifts that could serve as a sign of competence. Requiring these meta-narrative shifts is an ideologically produced difference, an example of the stigmatized vernacular.

The conversation between disability studies and folklore offers possibilities for greater understanding of how life on the margins is reconfigured. The importance of claiming Lucy and L as competent narrators is not to recuperate them as nondisabled or as not different, but rather to recognize how normativity works to stigmatize difference. I do not want to repeat the frequent mistake in folklore studies of recuperating and celebrating disenfranchised subjects as if such efforts might change the subjects' status or social conditions. My goal is not to diminish the difference in their modes of producing narrative. Instead, we can observe that Lucy, L, and their careworkers do co-narrate competently and that the source of the stigma, the failure to recognize the competence, is attached to other membership categories.[18] People with an intellectual disability, who rely on co-narration, and whose speech is otherwise marked as not "normal" are disqualified from recognition as competent narrators.[19] What we need in our model for studying disability is not only the tools for recognizing multiple normalcies, including the value of neurodiversity, but also the tools for recognizing ideologically produced differences and stigmatized vernaculars. The assessment of competency can be a hidden, unchallenged, overdetermined dimension of normalcy. The idea that an individually produced narrative is necessary for producing a sense of self is an example of an ideologically produced difference, an unsubstantiated assumption that serves to stigmatize individuals who rely on the co-production of narrative. In addition to observing the multiple normalcies that constitute cultural difference, disability studies reminds us to attend also to how normalcy is a gatekeeper creating margins and exclusions. For folklorists, the larger challenge is to recognize implicit normativity and the exclusions that follow.

Notes

1. Barbara Kirshenblatt-Gimblett's discussion of "value added" provides an important critical assessment of the role of value in heritage culture (1998:150).

2. For a discussion of paternalism in folklore, see Mullen (2000).

3. Instead, folklorists have more often referred to the distinction between passive and active tradition bearers (Goldstein 1971), a concept that could prove to be helpful for discussions of disability.

4. Disability studies scholar Lennard Davis traces the idea of norms through histories of measurement, and especially error, to the role of the Bell curve in identifying what counts as normal and abnormal in social practice and ability. His groundbreaking essay points out that the term *normal* came to prominence in a particular historical moment (1997:17).

5. See Devva Kasnitz and Russell Shuttleworth's extensive review of the scope of anthropological research on disability (2001). For examples of ethnographic studies of disability, see Frank (2000) and Groce (1985).

6. In her essay asking about the mutual benefits of cultural studies and anthropology, Anna Tsing recommends that "margins" serve as a "conceptual site from which to explore the imaginative quality and the specificity of local/global cultural formation" (1994:279). However, Tsing specifically states that margins are not only not geographical but also not "sites of deviance from social norms."

7. "Viewed in this light, folklore is an important mechanism for maintaining the stability of culture. It is used to inculcate the customs and ethical standards in the young, as an adult to reward him with praise when he conforms, to punish him with rationalizations when the institutions and conventions are challenged or questioned, to suggest that he be content with things as they are, and to provide him with a compensatory escape from the 'hardships, the inequalities, the injustices' of everyday life" (Abrahams 1968:147).

8. John Heritage, similarly, refers to "the competencies that ordinary speakers use and rely on in participating in intelligible, socially organized interaction" (1984:1).

9. Although I have not included a detailed sociolinguistic transcription, I have separated the lines according to pauses and have not used punctuation to render the exchange as an oral conversation rather than as a written text.

10. See Deborah Tannen's (1978) discussion of how expectations work in narrative.

11. Writing about mental retardation, Eva Feder Kittay says: "Those who speak do so in a language not recognized—and even demeaned—by those who speak in the language of the public sphere. Without a claim to cognitive parity, even those who can speak are not recognized as authors or agents in their own right. Those who cannot speak must depend on others to speak for them. Those who can speak find that their voice is given no authority. Perhaps there is no more disabling disablement" (2001:559).

12. Kristin Bumiller writes, "Antinormalization strategies potentially form the basis for a more far-reaching project whose aim is to shift the goal of the disability movement from simple demands for inclusion to a utopian vision of a society that values human diversity" (2008:980).

13. Some disability scholars put the "in" in parentheses, as if the discussion applies equally to competence and incompetence and to foreground the critique of incompetency labeling, but really, the problem concerns incompetence, not competence.

14. Disability theorists, especially deaf theory scholars, have called into question the centrality of speaking in communication historically and have identified the rhetorical positioning of speech (Brueggemann 2001).

15. For example, Arthur Frank developed a typology of three core types of illness narratives, the restitution narrative, the chaos narrative, and the quest narrative. In the quest narrative, "a character encounters a sequence of obstacles and gains wisdom and stature

through the process of overcoming these" (2012:47). Commenting on his earlier work, Frank writes, "My point was never to recommend one type as preferred" (2012:48).

16. For example, arguing against the deficit model, speech pathologist Jack Damico writes, "To become true experts in human communication, we must recognize the complex and interactive processes at work in communication and then formulate ways to describe and influence the construction and use of naturally occurring discourse" (1993:93).

17. For a review of research on the narrative production of the self, see Ochs and Capps (1996).

18. Harvey Sacks's concept of membership categories is particularly useful here. As summarized by Emmanuel Schegloff (2007:267), a category of people (such as people with intellectual disabilities) is assigned attributes (in this case incompetence in narration). Membership categories are fundamental to the process of assigning stigma, an issue I discuss more elaborately in Shuman (2011).

19. See also Dinerstein (2007) and Schweik (2007).

References

Abrahams, Roger D. 1968. "Introductory Remarks to a Rhetorical Theory of Folklore." *Journal of American Folklore* 81 (320):143–58.

———. 1993. "Phantoms of Romantic Nationalism in Folkloristics." *Journal of American Folklore* 106 (419):3–37.

Bauman, Richard, and Charles L. Briggs. 1990. "Poetics and Performance as Critical Perspectives on Language and Social Life." *Annual Review of Anthropology* 19:59–88.

Brunvand, Jan Harold. 1978. *The Study of American Folklore: An Introduction*. New York: W. W. Norton.

Bumiller, Kristin. 2008. "Quirky Citizens: Autism, Gender, and Reimagining Disability." *Signs* 33 (4):967–91.

Corker, Mairian, and Tom Shakespeare, eds. 2002. *Disability/Postmodernity: Embodying Disability Theory*. New York: Continuum.

Couser, G. Thomas. 1997. *Recovering Bodies: Illness, Disability, and Life Writing*. Madison: University of Wisconsin Press.

Damico, Jack S. 1993. "Establishing Expertise in Communicative Discourse: Implications for the Speech Pathologist." In *Language Interaction in Clinical Educational Settings*, ed. Dana Kovarsky, Madeline Maxwell, and Jack Damico, 92–98. Rockville, MD: American-Speech-Language-Hearing Monograph (30), 1993.

Davis, Lennard. 1995. *Enforcing Normalcy: Disability, Deafness, and the Body*. London, UK: Verso.

———. 2006. *The Disability Studies Reader*. New York: Routledge.

Dinerstein, Robert D. 2007. "'Every Picture Tells a Story, Don't It?': The Complex Role of Narratives in Disability Cases." *Narrative* 15 (1):40–57.

Docherty, Daniel, Richard Hughes, Patricia Phillips, David Corbett, Bremdam Regan, Andrew Barber, Michael Adams, Kathy Boxall, Ian Kaplan, and Shayma Izzidien, 2005.

"This Is What We Think." In *Another Disability Studies Reader*, ed. Dan Goodley and Geert Van Hove, 29–49. Antwerpen/Apeldoorn, Belgium: Garant.

Frank, Gelya. 2000. *Venus on Wheels*. Berkeley: University of California Press.

Garland Thomson, Rosemarie. 2005. "Feminist Disability Studies." *Signs* 30 (2):1557–87.

Goldstein, Diane E., and Amy Shuman. 2012. "The Stigmatized Vernacular: Where Reflexivity Meets Untellability." *Journal of Folklore Research* 49 (2):113–26.

Goldstein, Kenneth S. 1963. "Riddling Traditions in Northeastern Scotland." *Journal of American Folklore* 76 (302):330–36.

———. 1971. "On the Application of the Concepts of Active and Inactive Traditions to the Study of Repertory." *Journal of American Folklore* 84 (331):62–67.

Goodwin, Charles, and Marjorie Harness Goodwin. 2010. "Concurrent Operations on Talk: Notes on the Interactive Organization of Assessments." *Papers in Pragmatics* 1 (1):1–54.

Grove, Nicola. 2012. "Story, Agency, and Meaning Making: Narrative Models and the Social Inclusion of People with Severe and Profound Intellectual Disabilities." *Journal of Religion, Disability & Health* 16 (4):334–51.

Gumperz, John Joseph, and Dell H. Hymes, eds. 1972. *Directions in Sociolinguistics: The Ethnography of Communication*. New York: Holt, Rinehart, and Winston.

Haraway, Donna. 1998. "The Persistence of Vision." In *The Visual Culture Reader*, ed. Nicholas Mizoeff, 191–98. London: Routledge.

Herzfeld, Micheal. 1996. "Embarrassment as Pride: Narrative Resourcefulnesss and Strategies of Normativity among Cretan Animal-Thieves." In *Disorderly Discourse: Narrative, Conflict, & Inequality*, ed. Charles L. Briggs, 72–94. Oxford: Oxford University Press.

Heritage, John, and J. Maxwell Atkinson. 1984. "Introduction." In *Structures of Social Action*, ed. J. Maxwell Atkinson and John Heritage, 1–16. Cambridge: Cambridge University Press.

Hydén, Lars-Christer, and Eleonor Antelius. 2011. "Communicative Disability and Stories: Towards an Embodied Conception of Narratives." *Health* 15 (6):588–603.

Hymes, Dell. 1972. "On Communicative Competence." In *Linguistic Anthropology: A Reader*, ed. Alessandro Duranti, 53–73. Oxford: Blackwell.

———. 1992. "The Concept of Communicative Competence Revisited." In *Thirty Years of Linguistic Evolution: Studies in Honour of René Dirven on the Occasion of His Sixtieth Birthday*, ed. Martin Pütz, 31–57. New York: John Benjamins.

Inahara, Minae. 2013. "The Rejected Voice: Towards Intersubjectivity in Speech Language Pathology." *Disability & Society* 28 (1):41–53.

Irvine, Judith T., and Susan Gal. 2000. "Language Ideology and Linguistic Differentiation." In *Regimes of Language: Ideologies, Politics, Identities*, ed. Paul Kroskrity, 35–83. Santa Fe, NM: School of American Research Press.

Kasnitz, Devva, and Russell P. Shuttleworth. 2001. "Introduction: Anthropology in Disability Studies." In *Semiotics and Dis/ability: Interrogating Categories of Difference*, ed. Linda J. Rogers and Beth Blue Swadener, 19–41. Albany, NY: SUNY Press.

Kirshenblatt-Gimblett, Barbara. 1998. *Destination Culture: Tourism, Museums, and Heritage*. Berkeley: University of California Press.

Kohrman, Matthew. 2003. "Authorizing a Disability Agency in Post-Mao China: Deng Pufang's Story as Biomythography." *Cultural Anthropology* 18 (1):99–131.

LaCapra, Dominic. 1999. "Trauma, Absence, Loss." *Critical Inquiry* 25 (4):696–727.

Lévi-Strauss, Claude. 1987. *Introduction to the Work of Marcel Mauss*. New York: Taylor & Francis.

Linde, Charlotte. 1993. *Life Stories: The Creation of Coherence*. Oxford: Oxford University Press.

Lock, Katy, and Daniel May. 2009. "The Specials." http://www.the-specials.com/episodes/8.

Mattingly, Cheryl. 2006. "Hoping, Willing, and Narrative Re-Envisioning" *Hedgehog Review* 8 (3):21–35. http://www.ncbi.nlm.nih.gov/pmc/articles/PMC2987682/.

———. 2010. *The Paradox of Hope: Journeys through a Clinical Borderland*. Berkeley: University of California Press.

McDermott, Ray, and Herve Varenne. 1995. "Culture as Disability." *Anthropology and Education Quarterly* 26 (3):324–48.

Michalko, Rod, and Tanya Titchkosky, eds. 2009. *Rethinking Normalcy: A Disability Studies Reader*. Toronto: Canadian Scholars' Press.

Mitchell, David T., and Sharon L. Snyder, eds. 2000. *Narrative Prosthesis: Disability and the Dependencies of Discourse*. Ann Arbor: University of Michigan Press.

Mullen, Patrick B. 2000. "The Dilemma of Representation in Folklore Studies: The Case of Henry Truvillion and John Lomax." *Journal of Folklore Research* 37 (2–3):155–74.

Nelson, Diane M. 2001. "Phantom Limbs and Invisible Hands: Bodies, Prosthetics, and Late Capitalist Identifications." *Cultural Anthropology* 16 (3):303–13.

Nelson, H. L. 2001. *Damaged Identities, Narrative Repair*. Ithaca, NY: Cornell University Press.

Norrick, Neal R. 1997. "Twice-told Tales: Collaborative Narration of Familiar Stories." *Language in Society* 26 (2):199–220.

———. 2005. "Interactional Remembering in Conversational Narrative." *Journal of Pragmatics* 37 (11):1819–44.

Ochs, Elinor, and Lisa Capps. 1996. "Narrating the Self." *Annual Review of Anthropology* 25:19–43.

———. 2001. *Living Narrative: Creating Lives in Everyday Storytelling*. Cambridge, MA: Harvard University Press.

Ochs, Elinor, Ruth Smith, and Carolyn Taylor. 1989. "Detective Stories at Dinnertime: Problem-solving through Co-narration." *Cultural Dynamics* 2 (2):238–57.

Rafael, Vincente L. 1994. "Of Mimicry and Marginality: Comments on Anna Tsing's 'From the Margins.'" *Cultural Anthropology* 9 (3):298–301.

Rapp, Rayna, and Faye D. Ginsburg. 2001. "Enabling Disability: Rewriting Kinship, Reimagining Citizenship." *Public Culture* 13 (3):533–66.

———. 2011. "Reverberations: Disability and the New Kinship Imaginary." *Anthropological Quarterly* 84 (2):379–410.

Ritchie, Susan. 1993. "Ventriloquist Folklore: Who Speaks for Representation?" *Western Folklore* (1993): 365–78.

Rousso, Harilyn. 2013. *Don't Call Me Inspirational: A Disabled Feminist Talks Back*. Philadelphia: Temple University Press.

Schegloff, Emanuel A. 2007. "A Tutorial on Membership Categorization." *Journal of Pragmatics* 39 (3):462–82.

Schweik, Susan Marie. 2007. "Begging the Question: Disability, Mendicancy, Speech and theLaw." *Narrative* 15 (1):58–70.

Shuman, Amy. 2007. "Reticence and Recuperation: Addressing Discursive Responsibility in Feminist Ethnicity Research." *Journal of American Ethnic History* 26 (4):81–87.

———. 2011. "On the Verge: Phenomenology and Empathic Unsettlement." *Journal of American Folklore* 124 (493):147–74.

Smith, Brett, and Andrew C. Sparkes. 2008. "Narrative and Its Potential Contribution to Disability Studies." *Disability & Society* 23:17–28.

Tannen, Deborah. 1978. "The Effect of Expectations on Conversation." *Discourse Processes* 1:203–9.

Tsing, Anna L. 1994. "From the Margins." *Cultural Anthropology* 9 (3):279–97.

Watson, Nick. 2004. "'The Dialectics of Disability': A Social Model for the 21st Century?" In *Implementing the Social Model of Disability: Theory and Research*, ed. Colin Barnes and Geof Mercer, 101–17. Leeds, UK: The Disability Press.

Willett, Jeffrey, and Mary Jo Deegan. 2001. "Liminality and Disability: Rites of Passage and Community in Hypermodern Society." *Disability Studies Quarterly* 21 (3):137–52.

Williams, Val. 2011. *Disability and Discourse: Analysing Inclusive Conversation with People with Intellectual Disabilities*. Hoboken, NJ: Wiley.

CHAPTER TWO

Exploring Esoteric and Exoteric Definitions of Disability: Inclusion, Segregation, and Kinship in a Special Olympics Group

—Olivia Caldeira

Although there has been a nationwide movement to end segregation and promote inclusion for people with intellectual and/or developmental disabilities (IDD),[1] a recent investigation by the group Disability Rights of Ohio (DRO) argues that the state is doing little to support people with IDD becoming integrated into the community and that this is a violation of federal law. Citing the Americans with Disabilities Act (ADA) of 1990 and Congress's acknowledgment that isolation, segregation, and discrimination against individuals with disabilities continue to be serious and widespread social problems, the authors argue the state's overreliance on segregated residential placements, sheltered workshops, and facility-based day services is promoting further segregation rather than moving toward community integration (where people with disabilities are able to interact with people without disabilities). They also ask that, in addition to making supported employment in integrated work settings a priority, "integrated day services shall be designed to allow individuals currently placed in developmental centers or ICFs/IID [Intermediate Care Facilities for Individuals with Intellectual Disabilities] to participate in mainstream community-based recreational, social, educational, cultural, and athletic activities."[2]

This sentiment of integrating all activities, including recreational and athletic activities, is echoed by some in disability studies who argue the Special Olympics should be disbanded because it fosters negative stereotypes and promotes further segregation and stigmatization (see Counsell and Agran 2012; Storey 2008). My goal is to explore the concepts of inclusion, exclusion, and

segregation and the related stigmatization and stigmatized vernacular surrounding the Special Olympics by reconsidering the criticisms leveled at the
Special Olympics. Based on fieldwork gathered over the past five years with one
particular regional Special Olympics group, Ohio Special Olympics (OHSO),[3]
I ask whether the multifaceted relationships and understandings among group
members challenge us to look beyond the binary oppositions of inclusivity
and exclusivity to allow for an expanded definition of "folk group"—one in
which kinship is created through experiences of shared difference.

Inclusion: An Introduction

The topic of inclusion is a source of contention and debate for many in the
fields of education, policy, ethics, and disability studies and is a central theme
of this chapter because I'm interested in what is at stake when we talk about
inclusion, how this relates to the construction and perpetuation of stigma
and the stigmatized vernacular, and how categories of normalcy and acceptance are locally constructed. It is particularly relevant for folklorists because
it directly relates to emic (local or insider) and etic (outsider) understandings
of labels such as disability and normalcy, how labels are esoterically (relating
to one's own group) and exoterically (relating to an outside group) applied,
how stigma and value are attached to these terms, and ultimately how performance provides the stage for identity expression and management.[4]

On a basic level, the movement toward inclusion is a response to the dis-
criminatory beliefs that translated into very real and horrific practices (eugen-
ics, forced sterilization, institutionalization, to name a few) against people
with disabilities. Deinstitutionalization was intended to promote integration
in the community, but due to lack of funding, awareness, and adequate supports, many people with intellectual and developmental disabilities continue
to be isolated, segregated from the community, and unable to access the often
taken-for-granted rights and freedoms that are afforded those without disabilities. Segregation decreases the possibilities for interaction between people with and without disabilities, contributes to a fear of the unknown, and
increases the likelihood of misconceptions, stereotypes, and stigmatization.

In terms of education, inclusion refers to the Individuals with Disabilities
Education Act (IDEA) ruling that every child has a right to have an education
in the least restrictive environment. Integrating students with and without
disabilities from preschool through postsecondary education is a source of
considerable debate, and one in which I will only present some of the most
commonly used terms and arguments. There is a continuum of educational

services and student placement that ranges from full inclusion in general education settings without supplementary instructional supports to instruction offered in a hospital or domestic setting (Hocutt 1996:79). *Mainstreaming* is the term used to describe the integration of a child with his or her peers in a general educational setting for some part of the school day; *inclusion* means that "most children will be educated in the general education classroom for most, if not all, of the school day"; and *full inclusion* denotes that all children, regardless of their disability, will be educated in a general education setting (and thus there is no need for a separate special education placement) (79).

Proponents for inclusion argue that segregation limits the contact zones in which people of different abilities can interact, whereas inclusion provides increased opportunities for social networking and creating new friendships, in addition to ensuring students with disabilities have access to the general education curriculum (Mastropieri and Scruggs 2001; Sailor and Roger 2005). Disability studies scholar Michael Bérubé asks us to think about inclusion as an important means of teaching social lessons in addition to academics; conversely, he asks us to consider what segregation teaches nondisabled students: "*The 'disabled' are always other people. You don't have to worry about them. Somebody else is doing that*" (1996:205). Segregation is also criticized for setting a standard of lowered expectations that translates into even fewer possibilities for individuals with intellectual disabilities (Grigal and Hart 2010). Some of the most common arguments against inclusion cite insufficient funding and supports for teachers to give adequate attention to nondisabled students and the concern that the students with more specialized needs will not receive the intensive, highly focused, and individualized attention and support they need, thus causing them to fall further behind (Murphy 1996; Zigmond and Baker 1996). While these viewpoints concern the time children spend in school and school-related activities, they do not apply the question of inclusion and segregation outside of the school system and into the complicated territory of recreational activities for people with intellectual and developmental disabilities.

The Special Olympics: History and Criticisms

The debate about inclusion resonates beyond school and employment and into recreational activities like the Special Olympics because it highlights the tensions surrounding what it means to be a member of a group or a team, who defines the expectations and ethos of such groups, and in whose best interest those boundaries are maintained. The history of Special Olympics began in the early 1960s when Eunice Kennedy, who was disturbed by the unfair treatment of people with intellectual disabilities and the lack of safe and accessible recreational places, created a summer camp (originally called Shriver Camp) for people with intellectual and developmental disabilities (IDD) based on research claiming that by engaging in physical activity, people with IDD would have greater employment possibilities, better performance in school settings, and overall inclusion in the community. In July 1968, the first International Special Olympics Summer Games were held in Chicago, including over two hundred events incorporating track, softball, and swimming activities. In 1971, the Olympic Committee gave permission to the Special Olympics to officially use the term *Olympics* in the title of its organization; then, in 1988, the International Olympic Committee (IOC) endorsed and recognized the Special Olympics. Along with providing opportunities for sports competition, the Special Olympics began to include programs directed at providing free health screenings and some medical services to those in financial need (Healthy Athletes), numerous fund-raising endeavors, and SO Get Into It, a free program that teaches empowerment, inclusion, respect, and acceptance.

As of May 2013, the Special Olympics includes more than 4.2 million athletes and 70,000 competitions worldwide. Represented by the motto, "Let me win, but if I cannot win, let me be brave in the attempt," the mission of the Special Olympics is "to provide year-round sports training and athletic competition in a variety of Olympic-type sports for children and adults with intellectual disabilities, giving them continuing opportunities to develop physical fitness, demonstrate courage, experience joy and participate in a sharing of gifts, skills and friendship with their families, other Special Olympics athletes and the community."[5] To what extent this group's outcomes have matched its intentions and its ability to evolve with the changing viewpoints and policies that have occurred over the past forty years is debatable and warrants further exploration into how Special Olympics functions today. As a categorical group, does membership in a group such as the Special Olympics cause more harm than good because of the stigma associated with intellectual disabilities and how do we best approach an understanding of what group membership means to those most closely involved?

In his article "The More Things Change, The More They Are the Same: Continuing Concerns with the Special Olympics," Keith Storey (2008) offers a valuable discussion interrogating the Special Olympics and before proceeding with my research and analysis, I first must take into account some of his important insights. First, Storey criticizes the Special Olympics for being segregated, since membership is based exclusively on having an intellectual disability. Second, he argues it reinforces negative stereotypes by evoking sympathy and pity and contributes to further stigmatization based on the words often used to describe the Special Olympics athletes. The language used can be offensive, polarizing, reductionist in that it focuses on one's disability rather than on other aspects of their identity, not the language used by the athletes to identify themselves, and "lumps all the people in the group together in spite of their individual differences" (2008:135). Third, the events and activities lack a functional purpose and are often age inappropriate. Fourth, it is paternalistic and perpetuates a cycle of dependency because the coaches and volunteers are nondisabled and the athletes are the recipients of services rather than being in control. Fifth, financial resources promote corporations rather than assist in helping individuals with disabilities gain employment in the community. Finally, Storey states there is a lack of evidence-based research showing that the Special Olympics is effective in providing quality of life outcomes in the areas of physical, material, social, productive, emotional, or civic well-being. The majority of Storey's arguments fault the Special Olympics through its maintenance of segregation and exclusivity, with continuing to increase the divide between the individuals with IDD and the rest of society (what Goffman would refer to as "normals").[6] Based on these factors, Storey argues that the Special Olympics should be disbanded in favor of more integrated recreational programs that combat stigmatization and promote greater inclusion in society.

Building from the work of Storey and other scholars in disability studies, Counsell and Agran contend the "Special Olympics' antiquated lifeworld view of people with disabilities has largely resulted in outdated program practices supported by steering mechanisms that, altogether, run counter to today's emerging proactive lifeworld view of empowerment" (2012:253). They do cite the Unified Sports Program (a subsection of the Special Olympics) as a program that moves closer to a more integrated system as it creates partnership opportunities for people with and without disabilities to participate together in sporting events. However, they note that the Unified Sports Program is much smaller and geographically limited than the Special Olympics, and because it is based on pairing athletes of similar ages and abilities, it limits access to those individuals who require more extensive supports (253). What do integrated sports offer to athletes with and without IDD? In an article about a Unified Sports basketball team in Colorado, Andrea Cahn, the senior director of Project Unify, states that the interaction that occurs in Unified Sports transforms all of the students involved and creates opportunities to "pull back the veil of the unknown and make people real" (Frosch 2012). Whereas before participating in Unified Sports, some students with IDD felt alienated, they are now experiencing more positive interactions with their general education teammates through Unified Sports.

I question whether this setting and the ethos supporting it are really about normalcy because, as noted in the article, neither the players nor the crowds seem to mind who scores, commits traveling violations, or hands the ball to the opposing team to take a shot. This move from more traditional modes of competition seen in mainstream sports to the type of behaviors and norms valued in Unified Sports challenges the competitive component to sports and provokes different interpretations of what ideals and goals should be pursued, but it is misleading to equate this change in standards as being normal. Unified sports are intended to promote inclusion and normalcy, but in addition to questioning who remains excluded, do unified sports teams truly provide opportunities for normalcy, or is there an underlying premise of inclusion predicated on an inspirational narrative that, although well-intentioned, still borders on characterizing those with disabilities as mascots, thus reducing their access to full personhood?

If belonging to a Unified Sports team is difficult or impossible based on geographic availability and/or the severity of one's disability, and if Special Olympics is an outdated program that only compounds stigmatization and segregation of people with intellectual and developmental disabilities, why do some people continue to participate in Special Olympics? Is it a matter of a lack of other viable options, or is there something about being a member of this particular group that brings a different set of values and quality of life outcomes to the group that has yet to be explored? The debate about the Special Olympics provides us with an opportunity to explore inclusion and the role of the stigmatized vernacular in understanding inclusion (Goldstein and Shuman 2012). Folklore is particularly useful here for its understanding of group, how esoteric-exoteric labels are constructed and understood, and how stigma is sustained and contested. Storey's argument rests on the idea that a group that is segregated based on ability (or lack of ability) promotes stigma. In other words, the Special Olympics is not like any other sports team similarly organized around the level of competence of the players but instead is stigmatizing from the outset. Folklorists often study marginalized, disenfranchised groups, and a folkloristic examination of how groups perceive themselves and others helps not only to consider Storey's criticisms, but also to elucidate how the Special Olympics works from the perceptions of its participants.

Stigma, Special Olympics, and Folk Group Membership

Stigma directly relates to beliefs and assumptions about character, and by looking at OHSO, we can learn more about how people associated with a stigma perceive themselves and others; create, incorporate, or reject norms; and perform identity. Lerita Coleman cites a need for a multidisciplinary approach to understand some of the following: how the stigmatization of specific attributes is linked to maintenance of social control and power by some political groups, how some stigmatized persons overcome their discredited status, and/or how certain cultures are able to "successfully integrate stigmatized individuals into nonstigmatized communities and utilize whatever resources or talents a stigmatized person has to offer (as the shaman is used in many societies)" (Coleman 1997:229).

Folklorists have expanded their concept of what constitutes a folk group from the community bound by shared language, geography, history, and traditions to the complex dynamics described by Dorothy Noyes (1995) in her essay on folk group. Our desire to give power to stigmatized groups by labeling them as a unified community while recognizing the various factions, identities, and struggles for power that occur below the surface makes the application of a seemingly homogenous label of group a messy endeavor. Noyes follows the move from an emphasis based on text to that of performance and interactional analysis by exploring the work of Richard Bauman, who considers ethnicity, religion, region, occupation, age, and kinship (but not differential abilities) in his exploration of how texts and performances "differentiate the exoteric from the esoteric" (Bauman 1971:38).

Folklorists traditionally seek information from both those who are on the outside, potentially freer to talk and offer controversial or critical perspectives, and those on the inside, who might have access to the underpinnings and historical trajectories that have helped shape the group as it is presently. It might be assumed that those who are most vocal and able to articulate a certain self-awareness and awareness of the significance of what it means to be a part of the group are the cultural brokers, but generally speaking, (1) they are not often the athletes themselves; and (2) if they are, they are not representative of all athletes. As researchers, we are left in a type of quandary where a search for patterns elicits a sense of cohesiveness but also a recognition that each unique perspective is a reminder that this group is made up of individuals with very different circumstances, abilities, and perspectives—a warning to pay attention to the issues inherent in identity theory when applied to a stigmatized group. It also cautions us not to place too much emphasis on narratives and interviews as the predominant keys to gaining insight into someone's worldview, because communicative competence can exist through the performance of identity in ways that might not be possible through speech.

Anthropologists Faye Ginsburg and Rayna Rapp address the emergence of disability narratives that give people with disabilities and their kin a sense of belonging that moves beyond the biological family (2001:534). Ginsburg and Rapp's discussion of kinship adds an important dimension to folklorists' understanding of group insofar as it helps to account for the value of associating with a (stigmatized) group. They observe that disability narratives have the potential to offer insight into the lived experiences of what it means to be affected by disability and can "anchor substantial analyses of the social, cultural, and political construction of disability" as well as help us understand how notions of "rights, entitlement, and citizenship are conceived" (537–38). Rapp and Ginsburg are particularly useful because they reimagine the boundaries of kinship beyond the biological as people seek more information sharing and support. In short, my definition of this group as a folk group is based on what they define as a kinship group—both as recognition as part of a folk group and as shared experience, a dimension of tremendous salience for people that experience stigma:

> The cultural activity of rewriting life stories and kinship narratives around the fact of disability, whether in memoir, film, or everyday storytelling, enables families to comprehend (in both senses) this anomalous experience, not only because of the capacity of stories to make meaning, but also because of their dialogical relationship with larger social arenas. Indeed, the transformation of both emotional and technical knowledge developed in kin groups with disabled family members can foster networks of support from which activism may emerge. In other words, the way that family members articulate changing experiences and awareness of disability in the domain of kinship not only provides a model for the body politic as a whole, but also helps to constitute a broader understanding of citizenship in which disability rights are understood as civil rights.[7] (Rapp and Ginsburg 2001:545)

Rapp and Ginsburg suggest that the writings of the disabled and their kin offer an alternative form of kinship based on shared difference; this observation raises questions particularly relevant to my interviews. Many of the parents verbalize the support they receive through the other parents, but do the athletes feel a similar sense of kinship based on shared differences? Do the athletes find companionship and support through recognition of differences based on disabilities, or is the membership in the OHSO group the source of the kinship, without a necessary recognition of each individual's disabilities?

Before beginning to explore these conceptions of kinship, it is necessary to highlight some of the major characteristics that define OHSO. This group is not representative of all Special Olympics teams, even in the local area, but it is a team that operates specifically as a folk group because it is a geographically based group of athletes and their families who share common traditions and use the group as a means to socialize, spread information, reinforce values, celebrate rituals, and encourage physical activity. First and fundamentally, OHSO is a network of athletes, coaches, volunteers, friends, teams, and so on. Second, OHSO is a network that operates like a kinship network for the parents, coaches, and volunteers. Third, I've paid close attention to the other networks implicated in the lives of the individuals with disabilities—these networks are discussed at the Special Olympics events and play a significant role in their lives. It is noteworthy that OHSO, in this particular community, is the center and thus it is where I begin.

My interest in the Special Olympics began over ten years ago when I was introduced to OHSO. I became acquainted with many of the athletes, families, coaches, and volunteers and became a direct support provider for four of the female athletes in their family homes and also in the community. As a support worker, I was able to get to know each of the young women in-depth through participant observation and learned about their various personalities, strengths and limitations, (dis)abilities, and the struggles and successes associated with transitioning from high school to adulthood. From 2011 to 2012, I spent nine months in a different state working in a day habilitation center focused on helping individuals learn functional life skills and transition to employment and inclusion in the community. Unfortunately, segregation was the norm and it was overwhelming and frustrating to witness the social, cultural, physical, and economic barriers preventing many adults with IDD from having a successful transition into the community. I also noted that although several of my clients were also members of a Special Olympics team, they appeared to be less involved and had fewer sporting events, while the absence of valuable networks exacerbated the lack of information, transmission, and support that I saw as integral to OHSO. The accumulation of experiences led me to question how resources are utilized by traditionally disempowered groups, how the construction and performance of identity directly relates to locally specific conceptions of normalcy, and to examine the tensions surrounding inclusion as they relate to insider/outsider perceptions.

Methodological Concerns: Interviewing People with IDD and Their Family Members

One of the first issues I encountered in my research was the complicated notion of "informed consent" and how best to translate the project on a level more accessible to people with differing levels of competency.[8] The second issue I encountered was that many of the parents and guardians preferred to participate in the interviews without their adult children present. This could be because (a) they did not trust my intentions and were acting as gatekeepers to protect their children from potential stress or exploitation; (b) they wanted to speak frankly in private to avoid distressing their sons or daughters; or (c) they felt that their children would not be able to comprehend or contribute to the conversation and so did not feel it was necessary to include them. Whereas I would have liked to interview as many members of each family as possible, particularly the athletes themselves (to avoid replicating historical patterns of preferring the words of those in power over the often disregarded and devalued words and perspectives of those with disabilities), this was not often possible.[9]

The third issue that I encountered involved the actual act of interviewing.[10] Based on my prior experience with people with intellectual disabilities, particularly autism, and the effects of using declarative language (statement made without expecting response) versus imperative language (question demands an answer), the very act of asking a question can increase an individual's anxiety and shut down further positive communication possibilities. This notion of the imperative language requiring a correct response leads me to think about the interview format itself and how interviews connote other situations where individuals with disabilities have been evaluated and tested, often leading to further exclusion and stigmatization (although each individual might not link the causation between the two). Having attended multiple types of annual and quarterly assessments, individualized educational program (IEP) meetings,[11] and transition planning sessions and having performed various assessments (individual needs, daily living, life skills, etc.) required by my previous jobs, I find it difficult, if not impossible, for individuals with disabilities to not be aware of the invasive and potentially derogatory nature of many of the questions. In addition to the subject matter and wording of the questions being insulting (i.e., "Is the individual able to toilet themselves without accidents?"),[12] the individuals are being evaluated in areas where they may very likely have limitations and sensitivities to these topics (i.e., reading, writing, personal maintenance, etc.), and they usually are accompanied by at least one parent, guardian, or caregiver who not only answers the majority of questions, but whose authority trumps the answers offered by the individual with disabilities.[13] However, interviewing those closest to the individual with disabilities can be necessary to understand where he or she might require support or to articulate ideas, concepts, and provide stories that might otherwise go untold.

The fourth issue I faced was that the majority of the athletes could not articulate many of the issues of identity that we might expect or seek from typical interviews because they lack the ability to meta-narrate or articulate their disability. Because of this lack of conformity to what is generally recognizable as a reflexive personal narrative and the frequency of learned set phrases and responses I encountered, it is difficult to understand whether the individuals were trying to please whomever they perceived as an authority figure or whether they were communicating their true feelings. For these reasons, I chose to avoid any question or interaction that would reproduce the set answers they have been accustomed to providing, but also to take note of moments of resistance, canned speech, and disjunctures.

I discovered through emerging themes that these interviews provided the parents with a forum to talk about their experiences in a way that allowed them to give narratives that might not have otherwise been possible in a traditional interview—for example, what they find interesting about their child, how others have accepted or rejected their child, and where they have found support as their child enters different life stages. Whenever possible, if it wasn't already brought up in conversation, I also asked the parents what terms they used to talk about their child's disability in the home, with their children, and with other people in the community. This information helped me gauge what I could safely discuss when interviewing their children and (I hoped) would help me have a better sense of their child's level of self-awareness and how this relates to etic and emic labels and esoteric and exoteric definitions of disability.

Esoteric-Exoteric Framework for Group Identification

Disability is not a natural category, and it is interesting to look at how it is understood and used by those to whom the label is applied. It is something that is considered to be an etic label (medically informed) in that it is supposed to be externally observable and not value laden (as opposed to an emic understanding that is created from those observed and relates to their worldview) (Harris 1976). This is further complicated in disability studies as many have argued against the medical model as being deficit-based, whereas the social model focuses on the barriers in society as the disabling factors, and in response some have called for a new political/relational model for understanding disability (Davis 2002; Kafer 2013; Shakespeare 2006). The medical and social models are part of what makes the esoteric-exoteric framework more complex because they hinge upon different values and labels applied to those who are included in the category of disabled and thus excluded from those considered normal, which leads us to questions of power and authority in who determines such categorizations.

Folklorist William Hugh Jansen employs the esoteric factor in folklore to represent what one group thinks of itself and what it supposes others think of it, and he defines the exoteric factor as "what one group thinks of another and what it thinks that other group thinks it thinks" (1957:206–7). I categorize these components as Esoteric A (what one group thinks of itself), Esoteric B (what it supposes others think of it), Exoteric A (what one group thinks of another), and Exoteric B (what it thinks that other group thinks it thinks, or to put it another way, how it believes the other group feels it is perceived). I immediately encountered problems when trying to ask my participants to articulate who is considered the "in" group or the "out" group because the esoteric-exoteric model assumes stability in the categories of self and other. The OHSO group contains multiple layers and membership roles: the athletes and their parents, coaches, and volunteers have different levels of relationships and networking ties connecting them together. They are all part of the same group, but even among the group members, there are different belief systems, values, and communication styles and abilities. Not everyone is able to give an explanatory narrative defining their worldview, so it is impossible to find out what is in each individual's mind, but that does not deter people from trying and speaking on behalf of others.

Identifying who is an insider/outsider, the social circles that overlap and evolve, and who speaks for whom are just a few of the complicating elements encountered when trying to encapsulate the notion of the OHSO as a group. Even among the various Ohio Special Olympics group members, the following are some of the elements of esoteric and exoteric folklore that make it difficult to define clear boundaries of who is an insider or outsider within the group and what values or beliefs are attached to that status position: parents make assumptions about their own children and other people's children; the athletes have distinctive perceptions of themselves and the other athletes; and athletes and family members develop unique relationships with individuals who might have more fluid or transitory group membership (i.e., volunteers, support providers, coaches, etc.). These factors are just within the circle—when it comes to those outside of the group, there are many people who are categorized as outsiders (service professionals, teachers, mainstream peers, and the community), and different members of OHSO hold beliefs, opinions, and share stories and other elements of folklore (esoteric B and exoteric B) about them as well.

Jansen's model is useful for understanding what the esoteric-exoteric factor tells us about how people label themselves, how they think others label them, and how they in turn label others, but the awareness of labels is only one mode of articulation, and its usefulness is limited by the premise that everyone is capable of articulating and having self-awareness. My concern is that reflexivity, self-awareness, and the ability to communicate these concepts are inextricably linked to personhood, and thus a person is restricted from achieving full personhood by either not being aware of their disability or not having "a voice." In her research on competence and how individuals with IDD construct other selves, Charlotte Aull Davies argues that rather than suggesting low reflexivity is an inevitable result of learning difficulties, she suggests that it is "more likely due to social practices towards, and cultural attitudes about, people who have been so categorized" (1998:119). Since some of the parents told me that they do not discuss their children's disability around their children because they want their children to feel as normal as possible and not focus on the disability, it is possible that some of the athletes I interviewed did not have the language or experience of self-articulation surrounding their disability because they were not familiar with the discourse. However, not being able or willing to discuss their own categorization as disabled while still articulating their perceptions of others' disabilities signals a need for further exploration into the different ways in which labels and categorical membership are ascribed, accepted, or resisted.

Beginning with the first part of Jansen's definition of esoteric folklore (what I refer to as esoteric A)—what one group thinks of itself—I am interested in (a) how the athletes articulate the label of "disability," (b) how the parents view their adult children's disability, (c) how the athletes feel about OHSO, and (d) how the parents perceive OHSO. Several of the athletes spoke of being able to identify others as disabled based on appearances, behaviors, or differential abilities that served as markers signifying them as something other than nondisabled. Participants Patty and Matt said they can tell if someone has a disability just by looking at someone and seeing if the person uses a wheelchair. Patty said sometimes she can tell by the shape of someone's head and Lewis said he can tell by looking in someone's eyes. Other OHSO athletes spoke of behaviors as indicators of someone's disability. Nicki said that she knew someone who had Down syndrome, and when I asked her how she could tell, she said it was because this person talked to themselves a lot. This is one example among several where athletes identified someone as having a particular (but incorrect) disability, and I believe this is related to an abstract question requiring a response, to which many responded with a concrete example of a behavior that is observable but incorrectly linked to the accompanying disability. In addition to mislabeling, some athletes learn from their parents that someone has a disability, likely in an attempt to explain behavior that may be unsettling or distressing. For Patty, if someone is not able to control his or her emotions properly, displays anger or sadness for no apparent reason, or is "mean all the time," this marks him or her as disabled.

Participant Lewis measured disabilities in three areas: intelligence, behavior, and social interaction (how they are included in mainstream culture). He also talked about being disabled "sometimes," which pointed to the potential fluidity of the categorization of disabled as being something other than permanent or static. Using his own emic terms for disability, Lewis categorized people according to whether they were "special needs" or "regular ed" (included in mainstream educational settings). Lewis first began talking about how someone was special needs based on how well he or she could read. He then went into categorizing specific friends from the OHSO team and said that two of his teammates are "sometimes special needs"—for example, Nina knows math, when she takes her time, so this decreases her disability, and Ethan is able to memorize sports statistics, which makes him less special needs.

Lewis considers himself somewhat special needs (he made a gesture holding his thumb and forefinger about three inches apart) and said his friend Victor is only a little special needs (gesture of one inch apart) because he goes to college but sometimes has seizures and forgets things. His friend Charles, who cannot talk and is in a wheelchair, is not very special needs because he took regular education classes like American Sign Language, pottery, and woodshop, but his friend Henry, who is able to talk and walk, is a lot special needs because he is compulsive with food, eats until he throws up, and is loud in public places. Lewis also mentioned two other athletes who had bad tempers and didn't always follow the rules at Special Olympics events and practices, which made them more special needs than others. Lewis's categories of what it means to be special needs demonstrate a keen understanding of how normative behavior through following social rules can minimize one's status as disabled, as does inclusion in mainstream activities, but also highlights a thought-provoking understanding of both competencies and temporality. From an outsider's perspective, one might think that being able to walk and talk would signify someone as less disabled and having more access than someone who has difficulty with communicating and mobility. Lewis's perspective, however, reflects that being competent in areas such as demonstrating social skills is more relevant in terms of minimizing one's disabled status.

Talking about disability as it pertains to others is one thing, but asking someone about his or her own disability can be problematic. I have tried to follow Charles Briggs, who says "sensitive and effective interviewing thus presupposes awareness of the society's categories of speech acts and social situations and the rules for relating them" (1986:45). I noted that for the most part, the OHSO athletes were not forthright in discussing their own disabilities. Further, talking about something that contributes to someone's status as stigmatized can be perceived as invasive. I found that I was able to discuss individuals' disabilities with them and their parents by focusing on descriptive categories while trying to avoid value-laden terms (i.e., *normal*). Even using the word *disability* when speaking with some participants created tension, and it was difficult to find a language that was value-neutral. According to Val Williams, who discusses how the term *learning differences* is viewed during her group work on inclusive research, her colleagues with IDD hear this label as offensive and even mentioning the label can have catastrophic results (2011:189). This was apparent when I (OC) asked Nicki (N) about her disability after she had discussed other individuals on her team who have disabilities:

    OC: Do you think that you have a disability?
    N: Why are you asking? I just want to know.
    OC: I'm just curious.
    N: Yeah, I do. Yeah, I think I do.
    OC: What do you think it is?
    N: I forget.
    OC: Are there times when you feel like you have a disability?
    N: Sometimes.
    OC: When?
    N: I don't know when, but sometimes.

This was the only moment in the interview when she challenged a question and is significant as a point of resistance while also reflecting an underlying connection between disability and the stigmatizing effect it has, to the point where even mentioning it causes tension.

Whereas some OHSO athletes were unable or unwilling to provide a meta discourse about their own disability, others have grown accustomed to discussing their disability. When I asked Matt, "What is a disability?," he said, "In my case, disability means—I really don't know. When I first was born, I didn't know I had Down Syndrome. When they told my mom, I knew I had Down Syndrome." After Matt answered the question about disability, his mother asked, "When do you think you noticed that you had Down Syndrome?," to which he replied, "I was—I was looking in the mirror and I could tell I had Down Syndrome." We could be tempted to latch onto Matt's reflexive statement as an epiphany, where the way he sees himself collides with how others see him, thereby potentially offering us insight into Matt's inner world and his understanding of how disability is constructed. His mother became very animated and began trying to determine when this took place, so she asked what grade he was in, which school, and then tried to determine his age when he first understood that he had Down Syndrome by trying to match it to the teacher he had that year. The promise of a coherent narrative supporting Matt's claim that when he looked in the mirror, he could tell he had Down Syndrome, slipped away as his mother continued to question him to find out how old he was when this occurred. At first, Matt said that he was in sixth grade but then after further questioning, he said, "I remember having Down Syndrome when I was in first grade." For Matt, this could be an example of esoteric A as well as the point where etic and emic converge because a disability is something that a professional diagnoses and then informs the individual's family, but is also made apparent through reflexivity based on what other people observe and identify as signifying markers of a disability. It is possible that Matt is talking about an actual encounter with a mirror, or perhaps he is using metaphoric language to describe what he feels is the moment when he saw himself as others might see him and his outward features associated with Down Syndrome were first recognizable, or perhaps something else entirely. Rather than devaluing Matt's narrative for lacking consistency or coherency, I find it more useful to consider what these moments reveal about Matt's understanding of Down Syndrome as it relates to himself, Matt's mother's (and my) desire to learn the stories that reflect his inner world, and how Matt might have been performing the role of the storyteller to provide us with the narratives we so desperately wanted to hear.

When athletes did not articulate their awareness of disability, I spoke with their parents, who provided their own perceptions of how their children viewed their disability. Some believed their children were not able to be reflexive about their disability because they had known nothing different; in essence, if a person has always lived with a certain condition, how would they know what it would be like to not have that condition? Other parents said that they felt this lack of reflexivity and self-awareness was due to the very nature of their child's cognitive impairments, preventing them from communicating a meta-awareness. One couple stated that although they do not talk with their child about her disability because they want her to feel as normal as possible, they said they do see moments where she recognizes she is not able to pass as normal, as someone without disabilities, and they perceive this as causing her distress and embarrassment. Do we consider the parents as part of the in-group and makers of esoteric folklore or do these positions and groupings shift based on who is being compared and contrasted? Applying Jansen's framework, this is a point that doesn't fit neatly into an esoteric category because it is based on the parents' observation of their child's behavior that they interpret as a moment of seeing oneself as others see you, which they then categorize as sadness at not being able to pass, thus blurring the lines between insider/outsider, self/other, and projected notions of what each other is thinking.

Since I am interested in exploring insider/outsider categorizations, how this relates to inclusion, and the arguments put forth by Storey (2008) that the Special Olympics is a source of stigma and does not contribute to an improved quality of life, I wanted to learn from the athletes how they perceived their membership in OHSO. The majority spoke of it as being a place where they met and saw their friends. None of the athletes said anything negative about the Special Olympics; in fact, when I asked Matt, "Is there anything you don't like about Special Olympics?," he answered, "No, the people there are my family." This sentiment was echoed by the parents, who cited OHSO as being like a family where they received support and also found valuable information regarding jobs, services, and resources that they were unable to access through other venues (even from service professionals who were responsible for providing this type of information). Although it is an exclusive and segregated group based on disability, it also offers a sense of Rapp and Ginsberg's (2001) kinship model that might not be possible with integrated groups because this type of kinship is predicated on the shared experience of disability.

Although the athletes remained consistently positive in their remarks about OHSO, some of the parents criticized Special Olympics for not providing significant physical challenges, but these criticisms were outweighed by the kinship and belonging OHSO provided. One of the only criticisms of OHSO that arose from my research related to expectations and competition. Based on the premise that the Special Olympics is about improving one's physical fitness and challenging oneself to push one's limits through competition, some parents felt that there was not enough emphasis placed on vigorous exercise and that competitive standards were set too low for people to truly improve their skills and increase their personal best. One couple also admitted that although they had reservations about enrolling their daughter in OHSO because of the stereotypes and stigmatization associated with the Special Olympics, they discovered it had unexpected benefits in addition to regular exercise: social events to put on a social calendar and the ability to belong to a group of peers without an age limit, because although their daughter had been part of a mainstream team in high school, she had not developed any significant or lasting friendships with her mainstream peers. The athlete's father added that because of all the involvement of the group members, OHSO gives his daughter "the opportunity to succeed in whatever small ways that are provided. . . . I think that's been an eye-opener—pre-conceptions that

I brought to it, the hopes I had for my child after all, that this is a good thing for [her]."

Whereas the esoteric factor in OHSO that is fostered through events, rituals, and kinship can strengthen and help a group defend itself, the exoteric A aspect can also contribute to a sense of belonging, "for it may result from fear of, mystification about, or resentment of the group to which one does not belong." (Jansen 1957:207). While I did not come across much exoteric A or B folklore from the OHSO athletes, I did encounter exoteric A and B folklore about the Special Olympics from both the perspectives of the OHSO parents and caregivers and from those who were not members of the Special Olympics (but still held strong beliefs and opinions about what the Special Olympics signifies). I explore this in greater detail in another work, but for the purpose of this chapter, I highlight a couple of examples that support the idea that the stigmatization of the Special Olympics to which Storey and some parents refer coincides with Jansen's claim that the more distinctive or distinguishable a group, the more likely the occurrence of exoteric folklore about that group. The Special Olympics can be the butt of a joke, evidenced when President Barack Obama appeared on the Tonight Show with Jay Leno in 2009 and referred to his bowling skills as being "like the Special Olympics" (Storey 2008:134). Even when it is portrayed in a more seemingly positive light, such as the *Oakland Tribune* headline declaring "Special Olympics' Athletes Win Smiles: Races belong to not-so-swift, not-so-strong" (135), Storey would likely argue that it could never have value because it is always tinged with stigma. In this example, although the narrative is meant to be inspirational, it is still patronizing and does little to promote inclusion.

Since a sense of belonging is a major component of the esoteric-exoteric factor, and I'm interested in how this relates to issues of insider/outsider and inclusion/segregation, I looked for patterns of the exoteric A factor indicating how people in OHSO conceived of outside groups but ran into complications concerning who constitutes the other. None of the athletes I interviewed framed group membership using an "us vs. them" mentality, which could indicate that the majority of those I interviewed did not differentiate various group identities or that they did not regard outsiders as antagonistic to them. Two of the athletes I interviewed participated on some of their high school's mainstream sports teams in addition to the Special Olympics but did not claim a preference for one team over the other. When I asked Nicki what was different about her high school's swimming team versus the OHSO swimming team, she said that the high school team worked on different strokes than the OHSO team and that the OHSO team did not practice the butterfly stroke because it was too hard and she could not do it. For Tori, who was a member of her high school's track and cross country teams, it is unclear what social significance these experiences had for her. One of Storey's (2008) arguments is that while segregated recreational activities inhibit friendships and meaningful social relationships between people with and without disabilities, it must be asked whether inclusion and integration lead to greater possibilities for friendships. From what I observed with both Tori and Nicki, some of the mainstream students were more friendly and said hello to each of them, and while I do not want to minimize the effect this had on Tori and Nicki as well as their mainstream peers, it would be unrealistic to claim that these experiences led to equally reciprocated friendships. Nicki's mother had hoped the few friendships Nicki had made would extend beyond high school but saw that once Nicki's peers went on to college, the contact between the peers diminished. Tori's mother said that some of Tori's teammates invited her over for sleepovers and one girl from her high school wrote a prize-winning essay about her experience running with Tori, but Tori did not seek out friends on either team, and although she does continue to participate in social activities that her parents arrange for her, these are not things she would pursue on her own. Although both Nicki and Tori competed in mainstream and Special Olympics events and it would be interesting to learn their perspectives on the experiences to see if they experienced a change in their self-esteem or status based on participation in the different teams, both have a form of autism spectrum disorder that alters their expressive language abilities. Nicki does not articulate the reasons or preferences for group membership for the sake of being a member of a group, but she participates in rituals and traditions and wears the appropriate uniforms, and will say that she is a part of certain groups. Tori does not differentiate between "us and them" because her understanding of self and other is not typical (i.e., she often views Facebook posts on other people's walls as being directed toward her, has a difficult time understanding that people on television are not speaking directly to her, and also has concerns that if she talks about someone or discusses something that is meant to be private, that person or her neighbors might overhear). For Tori, everyone belongs to "us."

Regarding the esoteric-exoteric factor as relating to one group being antagonistic to the other, this is not a value that is reinforced by the coaches because although the Special Olympics does involve competition, the OHSO coaches do not motivate by emphasizing their athletes' superiority in comparison to other teams; rather, the coaches consistently teach the importance of teamwork and striving to reach one's personal best. If anything, OHSO is one place where there is a wide range of acceptance of difference, and this falls under the imposed norm of good sportsmanship. Trash talking and showboating are swiftly corrected by the coaches and reinforced by limiting an athlete's participation if he or she continues to violate the norms. Interestingly, sometimes the athletes are not sufficiently competitive and risk being disqualified for running in the wrong direction in a track event or touching someone to help them go faster. Although OHSO places more value on the social aspect—how to be a good sport and how to be a part of the team rather than on winning (which has been criticized by some parents)—there are some instances where the rules of competition take precedence, and it is noteworthy to observe how the athletes align themselves with what matters most to them at the time. An example of this type of disjuncture occurred at a track practice when the athletes were running the 100-meter dash. One participant, Janet, was heading towards the finish line, far ahead of her teammates, but before crossing the line she turned around and noticed one of her teammates was walking in last place. Janet stopped, ran back towards the girl, grabbed her hand, and they both ran forward together. When confronted by a volunteer who informed them that they wouldn't be able to do that during a real competition because they would get disqualified, Janet shrugged her shoulders and the two girls held hands and walked away. In this example, although the norms and rules prioritized competition, winning, and individuality, Janet rejected those values in exchange for reaching out to someone as a friend and creating a social bond that was more important at that moment than being the first to cross the finish line.

Conclusion: The Special Olympics as the Real World's "Other"

Exploring the values associated with the Special Olympics provides insight into how OHSO functions as a folk group that provides opportunities for learning social skills potentially translatable beyond recreational sports into places where the majority of people do not have IDD and/or are not as accepting of difference. Although the majority of athletes with whom I spoke did not place a significant amount of distinction between insider and outsider group membership, the parents were highly attuned to those whom they viewed as outsiders—and sometimes adversarial—groups, such as the school system, service professionals, doctors and medical professionals, and the community (particularly those unfamiliar with people with intellectual and developmental disabilities). This was reinforced through my observations of transition (high school to adulthood) meetings and Individual Education Program (IEP) meetings where parents and individuals with IDD were warned of the standards held by the "real world" and informed of the ways in which the child deviated from the norms upheld by "typical peers." Sometimes this meant that in the real world, things move at a faster pace and those who don't keep up lose their job; in the real world, employers and employees change, and just because one boss is accepting of people with disabilities, it doesn't mean the next boss will be. Also, in the real world, typical peers are self-sufficient and independently motivated to complete tasks (even the ones they find disagreeable) to the satisfaction of their employers. For those who require more processing time due to cognitive impairments, more maturity that comes from time and experience, or more opportunities to discover what motivates them and how to advocate for themselves, this abstract construction of the real world makes inclusion and acceptance even more difficult to obtain.

The esoteric-exoteric model provides a good starting point for understanding a stigmatized folk group such as OHSO, but it leaves open some of the central contradictions that sustain the group, especially the idea with which many athletes, parents, and Storey (2008) would agree: that involvement with the Special Olympics negatively stereotypes people with disabilities and yet the parents and athletes have created sustaining kinship networks around the experiences resulting from being stigmatized—the folk group is central to their lives and to their daily efforts to combat the stigma of disability. Storey and others would also argue that the Special Olympics does not represent the real world. The parents and some of the athletes agree that those leading OHSO sometimes prioritize the development of social skills rather than competition, but the "real world" of competition is itself an artifice, and the parents and many of the athletes know that they would never be able to "really" compete. Instead, having social skills can occasionally open otherwise closed doors. While I agree that more opportunities for integration and inclusion need to be provided to help combat the negative effects of stigmatization and segregation and promote greater opportunities for understanding and acceptance between those with and without IDD, I caution against completely disbanding all segregated recreational activities without first learning more about the benefits group membership provides to those who find kinship through the shared experiences of disability and stigma.

Notes

1. Although these terms are sometimes used interchangeably, developmental disabilities are those that are diagnosed before the age of twenty-two and can affect physical abilities, cognitive functions, or both. Intellectual disabilities originate before the age of eighteen and refer to impaired cognitive and intellectual abilities. http://report.nih.gov/nihfactsheets/ViewFactSheet.aspx?csid=100 (accessed December 9, 2014). In other words, all intellectual

disabilities are developmental disabilities but not all developmental disabilities are intellectual disabilities. The Special Olympics is specifically geared towards those with intellectual disabilities.

2. Penned by Kerstin Sjoberg-Witt, Kevin J. Truitt, Cathy E. Costman, and Samuel Miller, this Disability Rights of Ohio letter citing Department of Developmental Disabilities was published July 1, 2014.

3. Pseudonyms have been used to replace the names of the group and its members.

4. I am grateful to Amy Shuman both for sharing her current work and insights in this area and for her careful reading of this manuscript.

5. http://www.specialolympics.org (accessed December 2, 2013).

6. Goffman (1963:5).

7. See also Asch (1989), Bérubé and Lyon (1998), Kittay (1999), and Linton (1998).

8. The purpose of acquiring informed consent from participants is to give our informants a certain amount of assurance that we, as folklorists, will honor and respect their words, images, and perspectives to the best of our ability and afford them the opportunity to withdraw from the project at any time, for whatever reason. This process aligns with the requirements delineated by the Memorial University of Newfoundland's Interdisciplinary Committee on Ethics in Human Research (ICEHR). It also assumes a certain level of competence on the part of the participants, and although ICEHR recommends translating terms into those at a grade six or eight reading level for the general population, it was not always clear whether translating to a fifth-grade reading level made my project and its terms more comprehensible. Many of my informants were not their own guardians and did not have the cognitive abilities to understand abstract concepts such as anonymity, consent, or research, so although I translated my project into more accessible and less academic terms for those I interviewed and gave my university's consent forms to their guardians to read over and sign, the process warrants further attention and consideration.

9. This push to include the voices of those who have been ignored or silenced in the past has been encapsulated by the motto, "Nothing about us without us," but even Charlton (1998) admits that those with intellectual and developmental disabilities have been the minority among those represented by the disability rights movement.

10. I did not present questionnaires or surveys because I felt that asking open-ended questions regarding specific topics (i.e. Special Olympics, transition, what it means to be an adult, jobs, housing, relationships, etc.) would allow for a more natural, but semiconstructed, flow to the conversation where the interview could be tailored according to the topics and preferences of the individuals. This resulted in not every question being asked in the same manner to each participant, but it also meant that I had to take into account the context and individual communication styles and preferences of each individual.

11. An Individualized Education Program (IEP) is a written statement required by law to address the individual needs of a child with disabilities and addresses the following topics: assessments and evaluations of a child's current academic achievements, yearly goals, special education services, how much of the school day the child will be separated from children without disabilities, the steps needed if the child is to participate in state and districtwide assessments, modifications needed, how the child's progress will be measured, and transition

planning for those sixteen and older (or younger, if determined by the IEP team). http://nichcy.org/schoolage/iep/overview (accessed August 23, 2014).

12. This is taken from a Life Skills Assessment from a different state that is used to measure an individual's basic life skills in order to determine the levels and areas of support they might require.

13. Additionally, the parents and guardians fill out numerous surveys and are accustomed to being asked particular kinds of questions to which they've learned to tailor their responses according to the type of assessment, particularly to access certain services. Some are familiar with the need to downplay their children's abilities but conversely highlight their children's abilities where people might assume they don't have abilities. They would rarely have reason to exaggerate their abilities; this is not a population that passes as normal or mainstream (where people might go to great lengths to conceal their limitations).

References

Bauman, Richard. 1971. "Differential Identity and the Social Base of Folklore." *Journal of American Folklore* 84 (331):31–41.

Bérubé, Michael. 1996. *Life As We Know It: A Father, A Family, and an Exceptional Child.* New York: Pantheon.

Briggs, Charles L. 1986. *Learning How to Ask: A Sociolinguistic Appraisal of the Role of the Interview in Social Science Research.* Cambridge: Cambridge University Press.

Charlton, James I. 1998. *Nothing About Us Without Us: Disability Oppression and Empowerment.* Berkeley: University of California Press.

Coleman, Lerita. 1997. "Stigma: An Enigma Demystified." In *The Disability Studies Reader*, ed. Lennard J. Davis, 216–31. New York: Routledge.

Counsell, Shelly, and Martin Agran. 2012. "Understanding the Special Olympics Debate from Lifeworld and System Perspectives: Moving Beyond the Liberal Egalitarian View toward Empowered Recreational Living." *Journal of Disability Policy Studies* 23 (4):245–56.

Davies, Charlotte Aull. 1998. "Constructing other selves: (in)competences and the category of learning difficulties." In *Questions of Competence: Culture, Classification and Intellectual Disability*, ed. Richard Jenkins, 102–24. Cambridge: Cambridge University Press.

Davis, Lennard. 2002. *Bending over Backwards: Disability, Dismodernism & Other Difficult Positions.* New York: New York University Press.

Frosch, Dan. 2012. "Unified Teams Take Special Olympics Approach to School Sports." *New York Times.* http://www.nytimes.com/2012/02/13/sports/unified-sports-teams-open-doors-for-special-education-students.html?pagewanted=all&_r=0.

Goffman, Erving. 1963. *Stigma: Notes on the Management of Spoiled Identity.* Englewood Cliffs, NJ: Prentice-Hall.

Goldstein, Diane E., and Amy Shuman. 2012. "The Stigmatized Vernacular: Where Reflexivity Meets Untellability." *Journal of Folklore Research* 49 (2):113–26.

Goodman, Joan F. 1992. *When Slow Is Fast Enough: Educating the Delayed Preschool Child.* New York: Guilford Press.

Grigal, Meg, and Debra Hart. 2010. *Think College! Postsecondary Education Options for Students with Intellectual Disabilities*. Baltimore: Paul H. Brookes.

Harris, Marvin. 1976. "History and Significance of the Emic/Etic Distinction." *Annual Review of Anthropology* 5:329–50.

Hocutt, Anne M. 1996. "Effectiveness of Special Education: Is Placement the Critical Factor?" *The Future of Children: Special Education for Students with Disabilities* 6 (1):77–102.

Jansen, William H. 1959. "The Esoteric-Exoteric Factor in Folklore." *Fabula* 2 (3):205–11.

Kafer, Alison. 2013. *Feminist, Queer, Crip*. Bloomington: Indiana University Press.

Mastropieri, Margo A., and Thomas E. Scruggs. 2001. "Promoting Inclusion in Secondary Classrooms." *Learning Disability Quarterly* 24 (4):265–74.

Noyes, Dorothy. 1995. "Group." *Journal of American Folklore* 108 (430):449–78.

Rapp, Rayna, and Faye D. Ginsburg. 2001. "Enabling Disability: Rewriting Kinship, Reimagining Citizenship." *Public Culture* 13 (3):533–56.

Sailor, Wayne, and Blair Roger. 2005. "Rethinking Inclusion: Schoolwide Applications." *The Phi Delta Kappan* 86 (7):503–09.

Shakespeare, Tom. 2006. *Disability Rights and Wrongs*. New York: Routledge.

Storey, Keith. 2008. "The More Things Change, the More They Are the Same: Continuing Concerns with the Special Olympics." *Research and Practice for Persons with Severe Disabilities* 33, no. 3 (2008):134–42.

Williams, Val. 2011. *Disability and Discourse: Analysing Inclusive Conversation with People with Intellectual Disabilities*. West Sussex, UK: Wiley-Blackwell.

Zigmond, Naomi, and Janice M. Baker. 1996. "Full Inclusion for Students with Learning Disabilities: Too Much of a Good Thing?" *Theory into Practice* 35 (1):26–34.

CHAPTER THREE

Invoking the Relative: A New Perspective on Family Lore in Stigmatized Communities

—Sheila Bock and Kate Parker Horigan

The concept of "family" serves as a rich rhetorical resource in individual accounts of community trauma. Bringing together fieldwork materials from two independent studies—examining narratives of Hurricane Katrina[1] and accounts of Type 2 diabetes, respectively—this chapter highlights how family stories do more than signify the values and identities of particular groups. They also enable individuals to contest articulations of morality and blame in broader contexts of stigma. "Family" is not only a classification of a particular folk group or a descriptor of narratives' thematic content, but a rhetorical strategy employed by narrators in contexts wherein their reputations and identities are threatened.[2]

Since Mody Boatright's (1958) call to collect and analyze "family sagas," folklorists have generated valuable insights into the rhetorical work accomplished by telling family stories. Scholars in folklore and anthropology have examined how family stories respond to broader cultural discourses, particularly when these stories are shared by people who occupy stigmatized identities (Brandes 1975; Morgan 1966, 1980). In addition, following the performance-turn in folklore studies, folklorists began to look at stories as more than self-contained, static texts, focusing instead on how both their form and meaning can change depending on the teller and the context of the telling. Such an approach helped illuminate the personal factors affecting the meanings of family stories and the motivations for storytelling (Baldwin 1985; Zeitlin 1980). Other scholars have further explored the link between family and personal stories, bringing attention to the convergences between these two genres (Thomas 1997; Wilson 1991). Finally, folklorists have extended definitions of "family" (Danielson 1994; Goodwin 1994) beyond conventional ideas associated with the term in American culture (e.g., romanticized, heteronormative). These scholars have shown that "family" should not just be understood as a static entity that precedes family stories, but something that is defined, given meaning, and enacted through family stories and other forms of folklore.

Building on this important work, we aim to initiate an ongoing exploration of how "family" emerges as a narrative tool by which individuals refashion their relationships to communities and manage their perceptions by others, when those relationships are damaged by trauma, and those perceptions are constrained by stigma. While the topics of the stories we analyze overlap with themes that folklorists have commonly found in family stories, such as poverty and hardship, family migrations, natural disasters, and near deaths (Kotkin and Zeitlin 1983; Zeitlin et al. 1993), we look at these issues not merely as topics but as broader cultural contexts of stigma. Given that "family" invokes both self and other, referencing family in personal accounts of family health histories and community traumas allows individuals to position themselves in complex ways within broader contexts of community stigma.

Erving Goffman defines stigma as "an attribute that is deeply discrediting" (1963:3), clarifying that it is not merely the attribute that confers stigmatized status, but social consensus about how to interpret it. Goffman identifies three categories of stigma: "abominations of the body"; "blemishes of individual character"; and "the tribal stigma of race, nation, and religion" (4). To this last type he also adds class and writes that this category includes "stigma that can be transmitted through lineages and equally contaminate all members of a family" (4). The category of "tribal stigma" is particularly relevant for our considerations of narratives about family; family can be both the source of stigma and the discursive resource that people use to resist it.

Recognizing that "narrative is one means for individuals to negotiate and produce identities, sometimes in relation to otherwise stigmatizing characterizations" (Goldstein and Shuman 2012:120), we turn in this chapter to the narratives of people afflicted by stigma. In doing so, we are also answering Diane E. Goldstein and Amy Shuman's call in their special issue of the *Journal of Folklore Research* on the stigmatized vernacular. In suggesting a next step in stigma-related research, they write that while Goffman "considers how speakers take up a particular alignment, or stance, with regard to each other . . . he does not consider how alignment might produce, resist, enable, or confront stigma" (122). Our case studies attend to speakers' alignment with family members in their indexing of proximity to their relatives. In emphasizing their positioning with respect to family, these narrators are often reconfigur-ing their relationships as sources of strength rather than weakness. At the very least, they are reclaiming the right to define those relationships on their own terms.

"I got them babies on board": Hurricane Katrina

In the wake of disasters such as Katrina, official responders are faced with overwhelming demands for assistance. Deciding whether aid and empathy are warranted, and for whom, is a complex process with immediate and ongo-ing effects for disaster survivors. Thus, it is important to note that this pro-cess is shaped in part by stigmatizing discourses. In the context of Katrina in 2005, a prevalent narrative cast African Americans as responsible for their own suffering in the storm's wake. This narrative built on the stereotypes that African Americans are to blame for their own poverty and that African American mothers have excessive amounts of uncared for children. In one iteration, which is the focus here, this narrative emerged as a critique of fami-lies' failures to responsibly evacuate, therefore rendering them, in the minds of many people both watching and responding, undeserving of empathy and assistance.

Patricia Hill Collins describes how "dominant ideology suggests that Black children lack the attention and care allegedly lavished on White, middle-class children. . . . Such a view diverts attention from political and economic inequalities" (2000:84). She continues, "In this sanitized version of American society, those African-Americans who remain poor cause their own victim-ization" (84). Thus, Goffman's "tribal stigma[s] of race" and class overlap with "blemishes of individual character," and those belonging to a particular group are held responsible for the group's socioeconomic disadvantages. The general stigmatizing discourses affecting working-class African American families emerged in pernicious ways within the context of Katrina's aftermath in New Orleans. Furthermore, because of stereotypes affixed to urban African Ameri-cans, the stigmatizing discourses pertaining to post-Katrina New Orleans did not bother to differentiate among actual economic or social positions. This is illustrated, for example, by former First Lady Barbara Bush's assumption that "people she had seen while touring a Houston relocation site were faring better than before the storm hit" ("Barbara Bush Calls Evacuees Better Off" 2005). As a result, many people who may not be described—or more impor-tantly, may not identify themselves—as being "poor" are still judged based on prevailing narratives associated with that category.

As Susan Huckstep notes in her work on media coverage of Katrina, "Americans make distinctions between the poor who deserve assistance and those who do not. This distinction most often is determined by the degree to which poverty is attributed to . . . personal failings" (2008:21). More specifically, "Blacks are more likely than Whites to be portrayed as being poor as the result of personal choices. Black women, in particular, are portrayed as promiscuous, choosing to have multiple children and thereby remaining in poverty" (8). Suffering in African American families—especially those with multiple children—is rarely viewed as the result of exploitation or other circumstances beyond individual control. As a result, families with children who were unable to evacuate, as well as those who stayed by choice, were viewed through the lens of stigma. When their plight became public and their needs dire, assistance and empathy were slow to trickle in. This is in part because responders and viewers saw being stranded in New Orleans as indicative of bad individual decision making rather than as a sign of insufficient government planning, failing infrastructure, severe economic inequalities, miscommunication from public officials, or a number of other factors.

In a public opinion survey published in 2012, Lonna Rae Atkeson and Cherie D. Maestas confirmed that those who witnessed Katrina largely found its victims responsible for the events they endured. The authors report that when they surveyed respondents about "attributions of blame" for problems faced after Katrina, "the causal story that received the highest percentage of agreement was the failure to evacuate" attributed to New Orleans residents (Atkeson and Maestas 2012:80). This "causal story," with which "68 percent of respondents at least somewhat agree[d]," was in contrast, for example, to attributing blame to government response or to the severity of the storm (80). They also found that "positive valance images—such as victims reuniting with family and celebrating their safety or high drama rescues—appeared in only 20 percent of the segments on CNN and FNC [Fox News Channel], while negative images appeared in 52 percent" (54). Such a study, then, recognizes the stigmatizing narratives circulated by media networks and their power to sway understanding of causality following disasters such as Katrina.

Interestingly, though, Atkeson and Maestas classify the "non-evacuation" causal narrative in a larger category that they call "societal breakdown" (2012:79). For example, they also offer another instance of "societal breakdown," selected by respondents who felt posthurricane suffering was a result of rampant crime (79). By labeling residents' failure to evacuate as "societal breakdown," Atkeson and Maestas, as well as others who classify such a decision as a social rupture or anomaly, are missing something. The "failure" to evacuate was not seen as a failure at all by many who stayed behind, but rather as a successful demonstration of care for their family members, precisely countering the stigma of neglect and irresponsibility through which others interpreted their actions. Even while documenting stigmatizing narratives in media and public discourse, then, studies such as this one replicate stigma to some extent. In other words, what outsiders saw as breakdown or as careless, insiders saw as the ultimate act of intentional caring. Narratives of such insiders, survivors who did not evacuate and who did care for their families in the wake of the storm, illustrate both the stigmatizing discourses that constrain survivors as well as the rhetorical strategies by which they carefully negotiate their positions with respect to familial obligation.

In interviews conducted as part of the Surviving Katrina and Rita in Houston Project,[3] narrators frequently focus on family members while describing their experiences before, during, and after the 2005 storm. For example, in *Second Line Rescue*, Carl Lindahl reports that "Separation from loved ones is the most often-reported disturbing experience expressed by the survivors interviewed in the Surviving Katrina and Rita in Houston project" (2013:165). In these interviews, people frequently talk about mothers and children, often in stories expressing the care family members took of each other during extraordinary circumstances. In two examples below that are representative of this pattern, both narrators, who are working-class African American mothers, describe the lengths they went to in order to protect their children. Their descriptions of caring for children resist stigmatizing discourses characterizing low-income African American mothers as irresponsible. However, the survivors in these interviews do not romanticize their relationships with family; these narrators also draw the line in terms of family members caring for each other. These concerns reflect the obstacles that extended family networks potentially present in situations of crisis. In sum, as these survivors negotiate contexts of stigma, they resist totalizing narratives that misrepresent their connections to family members. Instead, they position themselves strategically with respect to relationships of family obligation, sometimes claiming a protective closeness and other times presenting a cautious distance.

The first narrator, Joan, contests stigmatizing discourses of irresponsibility and excess through her references to family members. She resists the discourse of irresponsibility by emphasizing the lengths she went to protecting her children and grandchildren, and she challenges the discourse of excess by setting boundaries around the family members with whom she shares a relationship of obligation. Joan is one of many New Orleanians who initially "sheltered in place" during Katrina, relying on previous knowledge of how to ride out hurricanes and a belief that the ride would be short-lived. After the levees failed and their neighborhood began to flood, Joan and her family were directed by rescue officials to locations where they were told they would find buses. Like countless others, Joan endured a long walk, then a longer wait, then finally, far too few buses for the amount of evacuees. In the examples that follow, Joan describes how she provided for her hungry grandchildren; how she fought to get them on a bus; and finally, how she risked her own hard-earned bus seat out of the city when she realized that her daughter and son-in-law were not on board.

First, Joan describes her general preparations as the family gathered before Katrina's landfall: "We had to prepare for the storm, as I say, we, I made sure we had batteries, search lights, matches, candles, water. I took all of the cooked food that I had in, in my apartment, so that we could have that to feed the children." After they have been stranded for some time, and food is beginning to run out, the children remain provided for: "And the children were not really understanding—they were enjoying theirselves, they had chips and cookies and they had their little toys, and they had food going, and they had cold drinks." Here, Joan emphasizes her role in providing food for the children, so they were sheltered from the danger surrounding them. Later in her interview, Joan recalls at length the dramatic scene at the buses:

> Well, I still had to get my grandbabies on board. So I pushed and I shoved, and I push and I shove, and I got them babies on board. . . . My daughter and mother-in-law was sitting on the seat. I gave her the children, and I looked back for my daughter and her husband. And when I looked, they were nowhere around. So I ran to the window, and I saw: they had done pushed them all the way back to the middle of I-10. They were sitting on the ground. And they were crying and just making sign, telling me, "No go ahead. Go ahead, save the children. Save the children." And I was beating on the window and telling them, "No! We got to stay together! Get on board, get on board!" And they was just crying and saying, "Go! Go!" So I push my way back off the bus, through all those people—I know it was nobody but God—how did I get back off, it was hard enough getting on. I pushed my way back off the bus. I ran to the middle of I-10 and I grabbed their hands, and I told them, "Get on, come on, get on." And we got back on the bus.

In the preceding quote, Joan emphasizes the extreme effort it took for her to get her grandchildren through the crowd of people, and then the subsequent effort to reach her children and get them to safety as well. She also describes the similar willingness of her daughter and son-in-law to put their family's interests first and "save the children."

This level of responsibility is not extended among all family members, however. When Joan eventually gets out of the city, her first stop is at the home of her son-in-law's extended family. She recognized she could not stay there because these people did not fall into her definition of "family," where that group demands care and protection. She explains: "I wasn't welcome, but I was grateful they still didn't say, 'No, you have to go.' Because after all, I was not related to them, and, space was limited. And food was limited, and—But anyway, they didn't say I had to leave." But leave she did, as soon as she could find alternative housing. Here, Joan indicates that though family networks may be extensive, they are not *excessive*. She is capable of recognizing, and others are capable of enforcing, the limits determining which relationships are bounded by obligation.

Another survivor, Patrice,[4] echoes the themes in Joan's narrative. Patrice also describes her extraordinary effort in getting her children on a bus out of the flooded city and then later describes how family members should draw boundaries when it comes to caring for each other. Patrice describes her experience with the buses as follows:

> So the man was—he told me, he said, "You can't get on the bus right now." I said, "What do you mean I can't get on the bus right here? The bus is right in front of me . . ."; He gonna tell a man, "Don't worry about her, she crazy." I said, "I'm crazy?" . . . [A]nd I said, "come on," and I walked my children right to that, that door, and when I got there, you know, they opened it, and they let me in, and that's when everybody came up, saying, "Oh, miss, you have to get off because I've got my baby with this, and I got my this," and I was like, "Go ahead, go head," and then finally I was like, "Uh-uh, I got to get my kids on this bus." So that's when we got on the bus and they brought us to Shreveport.

Here, Patrice faces opposition not only from authority figures, but also from other survivors who want her to prioritize their needs. She continuously insists that her own children deserve to be brought to safety. Despite the ordeal she had faced to get to this point, Patrice remarks, "it's like I didn't even feel tired or anything. I knew I had a task. I knew I had to save my children." Similar to Joan, once Patrice is out of the city, she resides temporarily in a number of places, including at one point the home of an extended family member. When she reflects on how she did not feel welcome at that home, Patrice explains, "At that point, if you couldn't accommodate, then I feel that they should have said no." Here, Patrice reiterates that boundaries are acceptable and even necessary in delimiting which family members fit within networks of obligation.

The discourses of irresponsibility and excess can have dire consequences for members of stigmatized groups. In the case of Katrina, the stereotype that low-income African American survivors were to blame for their own suffering led to less sympathy and fewer resources for those in need. As part of this stereotype, failure to evacuate responsibly was attributed to poor African Americans having large, unwieldy families. It is important to note, however, that according to many survivors, family obligations were in fact a common obstacle to evacuation during Katrina. Experts have observed this in retrospect as well, reporting for instance that "obligations to the extended family, especially the elderly, who resisted evacuation, inhibited many individuals and nuclear families from evacuating" (Eisenman et al. 2007:S113). By describing two kinds of family relationships, those of care and those outside the realm of obligation, Joan and Patrice negotiate stigmatizing discourses without pathologizing or romanticizing their family ties. Recognizing these values and limitations in survivor narratives can help avoid stereotype-informed decision making about who deserves assistance and can help to pinpoint actual concerns related to evacuating within an extended family network.

Viewing survivors' narratives in the context of stigma shows how the same decision—to stay in harm's way with family members—can have drastically different motives and consequences, depending on how it is viewed. When disaster response officials and the general public view this decision as confirmation of stereotypical beliefs about irresponsibility, it becomes an obstacle to much-needed assistance. When survivors view it as enacting appropriate relationships of familial obligation, it runs counter to stigmatizing discourses. Such a decision is entangled with stigma in other ways as well. For example, one study reports that because of perceived threats to the safety of drivers, a "physical barrier [to evacuation] was buses not entering the interior of the predominantly African American neighborhoods. This factor was reported to impede the evacuation of older individuals and those with disabilities, which, in turn, at times held up an entire family, who would not abandon those unable to walk to the bus" (Elder et al. 2007:S127). Furthermore, more generally, "Ethnic minorities do not seek assistance at the rate that white disaster survivors do. Stigma and mistrust may prevail when interventions are made available. . . . Efforts to create and use multicultural sensitivity in disaster interventions are only in the beginning stages" (Hall 2009:50). Thus, stigmatizing narratives influence both the provision of assistance and the willingness of those in need to seek it.

In the cyclical process of disaster response, officials take actions based on stereotype-induced beliefs. Either as a result of these actions or in anticipation of them, survivors—due to an acute awareness of the stigma that constrains them—take actions to protect those in their networks of care. As an exceedingly ironic result, they are seen as jeopardizing the health of their family members, hence confirming the narratives that prohibited their aid to them in the first place. Survivors such as Joan and Patrice offer a way out of this cycle: they are already creating—in both representation and reality—manageable communities for whom they are responsible in crises. If we attend properly to their narratives and consider how they position themselves in contexts of stigma, we will be better prepared to assist in overcoming the obstacles that these networks of care create and to help survivors draw from those resources on which they already rely.

This section presents just one way that the idea of family can become implicated in stigmatizing discourses and consequently can serve as a site of negotiation as narrators speak back to these discourses. The following section will identify another framing of family similarly connected to processes of stigmatization.

"Well, you know it runs in the family": Type 2 Diabetes

As the rates of Type 2 diabetes continue to rise in the United States and worldwide, public health officials now consistently describe this condition as a full-fledged epidemic. Amidst the extensive media coverage and health education efforts emerging in response to this epidemic, there are two prevalent narratives structuring much of the public discourse surrounding diabetes. One emphasizes the role of personal responsibility in preventing diabetes and its complications. Scholars have written extensively about how this framing works to situate individual choice as the source of blame, calling attention to how "lifestyle theories of disease tend to draw from constructions of sick or high-risk people as foolish, morally flawed, or ignorant" (Balshem 1993:24).[5] That is, the disease comes to be understood as a physical manifestation of problematic character traits.

The other narrative framing of diabetes focuses on the flawed nature of "culture," or the way culture stands as an obstacle to good health. Within this framing, to be healthy, individuals need to distance themselves from the unhealthy aspects of their culture, which are often transmitted and naturalized through the family. On the one hand, this framing deflects attention away from personal blame, which can be empowering for individuals. On the other hand, it has the potential to reinforce the experiences of stigma for people who are members of a pathologized group.

The people who come from the region of the United States known as Appalachia make up one such group. While actually quite diverse, this group is stereotypically viewed in much popular and scholarly discourse as being marked by "passive victimization at the hands of fate" (Billings 1999:11). In his critique of such stereotypical perceptions, Billings points to one representative example in which a social scientist described the "traumatized culture" of Appalachians that is passed on from generation to generation, characterized by "a numbness of spirit," "a sense of resignation," and "a retreat into fatalism" (Cattell-Gordon 1990:55). As rates of lifestyle diseases such as diabetes have risen within Appalachian communities, the role of Appalachian cultural traditions and character traits in this health crisis have often been foregrounded, situating Appalachian culture as a threat to health.[6]

As in the interview data from the SKRH project presented in the previous section, within interviews conducted with people who had, or were at risk for, diabetes, references to family were prevalent.[7] The most prominent theme within these references is the idea that diabetes runs in the family, and narrators use references to family histories to negotiate the stigmatizing discourses surrounding diabetes. One such narrator is Gail,[8] a fifty-one-year-old woman with a family history of diabetes.

Gail's mother's family was originally from rural West Virginia, and her mother moved to Indianapolis as part of the larger migration of Appalachians northward into urban areas to work in the automobile industry. When talking about growing up in Indianapolis, she recounted her own and her family members' experiences of being treated badly by schoolteachers and physicians because of her Appalachian background, being told, for example, "you people don't seem to understand." As a child, Gail would travel with her mother to West Virginia to visit her extended family. As an adult, Gail moved to Columbus, Ohio, with her female partner, who was raised Jewish, and converted to Judaism. Together, they have a young daughter, though she is now separated from the partner. Gail does not have diabetes herself, though several women in her family do, including her mother and her maternal aunts, so she considers herself to be at risk for getting diabetes in the future.

Gail's experiences are neither representative of people who have a family history of diabetes nor of Appalachians' experiences more broadly. Rather, the way she frames her family history is representative of patterns found across multiple interviews, as her interview richly illustrates strategic negotiation of the pathologizing discourses of individual responsibility and flawed culture in the context of a stigmatized family legacy. As Gail discusses her family legacy of diabetes, she employs two representative rhetorical strategies of de-stigmatization: externalization, which involves positioning blame outside the individual, and reorientation, which involves offering a new way of viewing traits that members of a group share. Using these strategies, she positions both her family members and herself in ways that speak back to broader discourses of stigma.

To understand Gail's strategy of externalization, consider the following excerpt from her interview:

> We also had this very bizarre—this is odd—but we have a huge family history of amputation, and a couple of the women lost a lower leg to diabetes, but bizarrely, I have a bunch of uncles who are amputees. It's not bizarre if you're from that culture, but they worked on the trains. You could work in the mines and you'd get black lung, and I had one uncle that had the oxygen tank with the little tubes. And some of them joined the army and got out, because they didn't want to work in the mines. The other thing you could do is you could work on the coal cars, and those cars weigh tons. They'd climb around on those moving trains, and if you worked there long enough, you will fall off and be run over by a train. For some reason, none of my uncles were cut in half or lost a head or an arm—they all lost a leg. So I actually have, like, 3 or 4 uncles, one of whom had no legs, and the others had one leg, and they'd all fallen off the back of a train and had a train run over them. And they all had artificial legs.
>
> So, I had these 3 or 4 amputee uncles, and then I had a couple of aunts that lost a leg to diabetes, so I kind of had this feeling like we have this family legacy of losing a leg. Crutches were a completely normal thing in my mom's extended family. Like, people hobbling.
>
> I have a story that's probably useless for your [research], but I was staying, visiting my mom's house where she grew up, 2 or 3 times, and it was literally like a shack. It was long, divided into two rooms. There was a main part and there were two bunk rooms—what had been the girls' room and the boys' room, and all these uncles were back visiting because my mom was there. Well, I had no idea, I was only 5 or 6 at the time, and I didn't know they'd all lost their leg. They all limped, but the leg was dressed. They had pants and a white sock and a black shoe. They all would take off their leg, and the leg was dressed, and they'd lay the legs on the floor to go to bed. So, I got up in the middle of the night to go to the outhouse, because they didn't have indoor plumbing, and my mom told me to go out through my uncles' room and go out through the back, and I came into this room and there's all these dressed legs laying on the floor! I have this surrealistic vision of legs everywhere, but there were probably 2 or 3. But of course, I'd never heard of an artificial leg, so I was just screaming! My mom was like, "Oh, it's just your uncles' legs [laughing]."

Later on in her interview, as she discusses how well her mother and aunts took care of their diabetes, she refers back to this legacy:

> Well, I would say depending on the personality, my mom and aunts had a wide spectrum of how seriously they took their diabetes and how well they did what the doctor asked them to do, and how they changed their lives. I think a couple of the aunts managed it correctly. I would think that they were the aunts that had the more supportive husbands, and the less troubled marriages, which is also a big legacy in our family. They tended to marry kind of difficult men, or men that had their legs cut off by the railroad. Money problems and stuff. So, I think a couple of the aunts had made good marriages, and so I think they had a supportive spouse and a less stressful daily life, and I think those, they took their medicine like they were supposed to, and were careful about what they ate.

Exemplifying the strategy of externalization, she situates her aunts' and uncles' lost legs as part of the same "family legacy," offering a broader context within which to understand her aunts' diabetes-related complications. She also draws connections between her family's experiences and cultural experiences. That is, this is not an issue that is unique either to her individual family members or to her individual family. Additionally, through the contextual information she offers, such as the lack of job opportunities, she attributes the men's amputations to economic factors and occupational hazards beyond their control. Her identification of the occupational hazards of working in the mines further diverts responsibility for the amputations away from her uncles. It was just part of the job, like black lung. She reinforces this broader idea of economic disadvantage by highlighting poverty in setting the scene of her personal narrative about her discovery of this family legacy. Finally returning once again to the legacy of diabetes and its complications for the women in her family, she draws a clear connection between the men's amputations, the familial stress due to resulting financial difficulties, and her aunts' abilities to take good care of their diabetes. In other words, the poor diabetes management practiced by some of her aunts was highly influenced by stress, which is directly attributable to the lack of economic opportunities she referenced before. Gail's story, then, works to contextualize the prevalence of diabetes-related amputations in her family by situating this legacy within broader structures of inequality, in effect destabilizing the stigmatizing discourses by externalizing the sources of blame.

Of course, there are limits to this strategy of externalization, especially for groups like Appalachians, whose public image is linked to the problematic (and inherited) cultural characteristics of resignation and fatalism, which in turn reinforces the stigmatizing narrative that the prevalence of lifestyle illnesses within this population is the result of contagious group affiliations. By filtering these "inherited" feelings of fatalism through the lens of her own experiences, Gail offers a reoriented way of viewing (and ultimately valuing) them. For example, in her discussion of how her mother and her aunts responded to the prevalence of diabetes and diabetes-related complications in her family, Gail explains how she saw herself as inheriting the feeling of inevitability shared by these family members:

> I think that people saw it as inevitable. I think of it as inevitable for myself. I'm 51, and I don't have it yet, but I feel like I—and the doctor told me years ago that at some point, you'll get it. From that many people in your family, when the women in your family get it. It's sort of like the breast cancer thing, your probability is so high, and I try to keep my weight down because we now know that with Type 2, it's how much body weight you carry that's the primary thing, so I work hard to keep it down. But I have a feeling of inevitability, and I think I must have inherited it from them. My thought's always been if I can hold it off until, like, 60. Since I'm 51, I think if I can become only pre-diabetic in my late 50s or slightly diabetic and I can manage it with my diet, then maybe I wouldn't have to take insulin until maybe I'm in my 70s or something, and then maybe I'll have died of something else, or maybe I won't care as much. I think it must come from that. I think they've [the women in my family] had an inevitable feeling. They'd call each other on the phone and say, "The doctor says I've got the sugar." And they'd be like, "Well, you know it runs in the family."

In her explanation of her views on her own health, she identifies her young daughter as her primary motivation for staying healthy and living longer. Despite this strong motivation, she describes the inherited "feeling of inevitability" as something she consciously has to push back against in her attempts to adopt a healthy lifestyle.

It is notable that she does not deny the existence of resignation within her family; she frames this inheritance as often standing in the way of making healthy choices, which might appear to validate the stigmatizing discourses about the flawed nature of Appalachian culture. At the same time, she shares experiences that highlight the role this cultural inheritance has played in other aspects of her life. Consider the following example, in which she recounts an experience where she thought she was dying:

> I had my own medical crisis, which is everybody thought I had a heart attack, and I didn't have one, but it felt like one. . . . I really thought I was going to

die. . . . So for a couple of days, I walked around thinking, like an aftershock from an earthquake, wondering when it's going to get me. In a way it was kind of tied to—okay, this is what happens to women in our family. We all just die young. Maybe it's my time. And maybe there is some comfort, because they all passed kind of early, I didn't feel so cheated. Like, I didn't think it's not fair, I'm only 49. Sometimes it happens. And also because of, I think, the religious background. Oddly, both the Appalachian and the Jewish culture have that unfairness of life aspect. That it cuts down some people in youth and some people live to old age, and it's a religious theme for cultures. Like, why is that, why is it so unfair, and accepting the unfairness in both religions is huge, so I did pretty good with it. . . . And my dad was not like that, and he's not from that culture. My dad, the last week when he knew he was dying, my sister said he was terrified. He couldn't sleep, he had to have sedatives. . . . So, I'm kind of grateful to be from my mom's side. . . . It's my fate, and I accept it. . . . In a weird way, the fatalism and the religiosity is kind of a mixed bag.

Here, Gail identifies connections between the religion she was raised in and the one she converted to, in effect highlighting how feelings of resignation are not unique to Appalachian culture. She also presents these feelings of inevitability as something for which she is ultimately grateful. She further emphasizes the positive value of the traits she inherited from her mother's side of the family by contrasting her experience with her father's experience of dying, attributing this difference to the fact that "he's not from that culture." Her reorientation, or revaluing, of her family inheritance does not completely disregard the challenges that they can bring. By recognizing her family inheritance as "kind of a mixed bag," she identifies it as something she both wishes to align hers7elf with and distance herself from. As with the narrators who recounted their experiences trying to leave New Orleans after Hurricane Katrina, Gail (and others) neither fully romanticizes nor pathologizes the role of family in her presentation of self. Gail shows how responses to stigma can be more complex than mere opposition, instead involving a good deal of negotiation.

Scholars and practitioners from a range of disciplines have urged healthcare professionals working with patients with family histories of illness to pay attention to how family beliefs can influence individuals' perceptions of personal risk.[9] For example, nursing scholar Melissa Scollan-Koliopoulos asserts that "If previous generations had a relentless, progressive course, such as a fatal outcome or disability related to diabetes, the patient will be left with a legacy of hopelessness about the condition (Rolland 1999). This concept is vital when working with an individual with a multigenerational transmission of diabetes" (Scollan-Koliopoulos 2004:226). Such scholarship demonstrates awareness that qualitative interviews are useful tools for understanding health beliefs, that personal health beliefs do not exist in a vacuum, and that beliefs shared within families can influence how individuals respond to health concerns. However, professionals engaged in this important work could benefit from more explicit attention to negotiations in people's articulations of their beliefs, especially when they are shared within contexts of stigma. The extent to which healthcare professionals recognize how these broader contexts of stigma are shaping individuals' beliefs and experiences (as well as how individuals are responding to them) can greatly affect relationships they develop with their patients.

Conclusion

Narrators use the concept of family as a rhetorical strategy to negotiate and contest stigmatizing discourses in these two contexts of disaster and illness— contexts that affect both individuals and the groups to which they belong. The parallels in these studies show how stories about family are one of the narrative means by which people confront stigma. In both contexts, not only are people's lives thrown into flux, but the perceptions by which others evaluate their lives take on critical consequences. These are both cases where those with the power to distribute resources, whether through health care or emergency assistance, frequently view the recipients of those resources as undeserving. Thus, stigma creates practical obstacles for both of these groups. In our examples, people affected by illness and disaster confront the obstacle of stigma by constructing their plight as greater than themselves: they make connections to family histories to show how their diabetes is not only the result of individual choices, and they emphasize their care for family members to show how they made morally sound decisions during Katrina. Moreover, the recourse to family in these accounts is not random. In both cases, outsiders and dominant discourses construct "family" as a dangerous or unruly burden. Family relationships are invoked in these personal narratives, then, in response to the way families are implicated in the stigmatizing discourses. In bringing these studies together, we intend to initiate ongoing attention to a different dimension of family narratives in folklore scholarship; we also envision that studies such as ours will have productive practical applications for professionals working within similar contexts of stigma.

Whereas family lore has traditionally referred in folklore studies to narratives shared *within* families, our respective studies focus on individual narrators who share their stories with someone outside of their families. This raises questions of interest to us and no doubt to other folklorists as well. For example, we do not know whether these particular narratives are shared among family members, nor do we know whether they are part of these narrators' repertoires, and if so, how they repeat or differ in other contexts of performance.[10] Although we recognize the value in such knowledge and hope that future research enables its discovery, these are not the questions that have guided this particular inquiry. In fact, stories told within families would not serve our purposes here of determining how folklorists and others might practically impact the fields of healthcare and disaster recovery; here, we are interested in how family is presented to others, not how it is constructed within itself. Therefore, we hope others interested in family folklore will consider this expanded arena of attention, including stories people tell *about* their families and interpreting how those stories are used as strategic resources.

We also anticipate that studies such as ours may be instructive for folklorists or other scholars doing qualitative research in contexts of stigma. Because we noted a pattern among our independent data and then across our two research areas, we have been able to identify family as one salient topic that narrators use in productive ways. Even in our two case studies, though, differences emerge with respect to how narrators position themselves, for example, focusing more on historical legacies of health or contemporary networks of care. Therefore, we expect that in other cases, rhetorical recourse to stories about family will be similarly unique and context-specific. However, we hope that researchers working in contexts of stigma will attend to this type of family narrative, discovering what type of work it is doing for narrators in other situations. We also imagine that narrative recourse to other groups, such as neighborhood or regional affiliations, could be similarly employed by narrators in cases where those group identities are entwined with stigmatizing discourses that constrain narrators and affect their daily lives. We suggest, though, that rather than look to match narrators' words with anticipated stereotypes, researchers allow narrators' own emphases to guide identification of significant categories.

Finally, we are hopeful about the practical applications for studies like this one. When individuals and families are implicated in stigmatizing discourses, it is important to recognize that this context of stigma can shape the ways in which people articulate their beliefs and experiences (especially when talking to someone they do not know well, such as a healthcare provider, disaster response official, or researcher). Therefore, interviews that elicit information about the relationship between individual and family beliefs or experiences need to attend to additional contexts as well, and these contexts are often signaled by the patterns that emerge in narratives. We have outlined here how interviewers might attend to speakers' interactions with larger contexts by paying attention to strategies of positioning, such as externalization and reorientation in the case of diabetes, and claiming or limiting relationships of obligation in the case of Katrina. Healthcare providers, disaster responders, and researchers would benefit greatly from being mindful of how individuals recount their experiences in response to broader stigmatizing discourses. Ultimately, we believe that professionals working with people in contexts of stigma can work more effectively when they understand both the context and how those with whom they work are already navigating within it.

Notes

1. Hurricane Katrina struck the Gulf Coast of the United States in August 2005. Official estimates report that more than 1,800 people in the affected area died, more than one million people lost their homes, and hundreds of thousands of people were displaced, many never to return.

2. We presented key ideas in this chapter at the 2014 Annual Meeting of the Western States Folklore Society. We are grateful to those who attended our presentation and provided feedback that has been influential as we prepared this chapter for publication.

3. Surviving Katrina and Rita in Houston (SKRH) is a documentation project created by Carl Lindahl and Pat Jasper, wherein hurricane survivors displaced to Houston were hired and trained to interview their fellow evacuees. http://www.survivingkatrinaandrita.dgs-sites.com.

4. Pseudonym.

5. See also Brandt and Rozin (1997); Broom and Whittaker (2004); Crawford (1977; 1980); and Lupton (1995).

6. For example, a *Salon* article reporting on diabetes in Appalachia foregrounds culture as an obstacle to effective treatment, highlighting that, "In Appalachia, fighting diabetes means *battling a culture* where even vegetables tend to be covered in bacon fat" (Browning 2012; emphasis added). The article also references "a deep-seated fatalism" as a major barrier toward treating diabetes effectively.

7. These interviews were conducted as part of a larger fieldwork-based project carried out in Columbus, Ohio, between 2006 and 2009 that examined discourses of "culture" in vernacular and institutional framings of Type 2 diabetes.

8. Pseudonym.

9. See Lindenmeye et al. (2008); Richards (1997); Walter and Emery (2005); Walter et al. (2004); Werner-Lin (2007); and Werner-Lin and Gardner (2009). For the most part, the perspectives of folklorists have not been represented in this work. One notable exception is the partnership formed between the American Folklife Center, the Institute for Cultural Partnerships, the American Society of Human Genetics, and the Genetic Alliance in 2005 in order to develop a Family History Tool. The goal of this project was "to increase awareness

and understanding of ways family history may influence personal health and [to] use an oral history approach to help family members gather health-related information from each other" (Family History Tool Project).

10. Elsewhere, each of us has brought these types of questions to bear on our research data, analyzing multiple presentations of the same personal narrative about Type 2 diabetes and Hurricane Katrina, respectively. These analyses, however, did not give focused attention to the idea of "family" we are suggesting here (Bock 2012; Horigan 2013).

References

Atkeson, Lonna Rae, and Cherie D. Maestas. 2012. *Catastrophic Politics: How Extraordinary Events Redefine Perceptions of Government*. New York: Cambridge University Press.

Baldwin, Karen. 1985. "'Woof!': A Word on Women's Roles in Family Storytelling." In *Women's Folklore, Women's Culture*, ed. Rosan A. Jordan and Susan J. Kalčik, 149–62. Philadelphia: University of Pennsylvania Press.

Balshem, Martha. 1993. *Cancer in the Community: Class and Medical Authority*. Washington, DC: Smithsonian Institution Press.

Bamberg, Michael G. W. 1997. "Positioning Between Structure and Performance." *Journal of Narrative and Life History* 7 (1–4):335–42.

"Barbara Bush Calls Evacuees Better Off." *New York Times*, September 7, 2005. http://www.nytimes.com/2005/09/07/national/nationalspecial/07barbara.html?_r=0.

Billings, Dwight B. 1999. "Introduction." In *Back Talk from Appalachia: Confronting Stereotypes*, ed. Dwight B. Billings, Gurney Norman, and Katherine Ledford, 3–20. Lexington: University Press of Kentucky.

Boatright, Mody C. 1958. "The Family Saga as a Form of Folklore." In *The Family Saga and Other Phases of American Folklore*, ed. Mody C. Boatright, Robert B. Downs, and John T. Flannagan, 1–19. Urbana: University of Illinois Press.

Bock, Sheila. 2012. "Toward a Performance Approach to African American Personal Narratives about Diabetes." *Western Journal of Black Studies* 36 (4):276–88.

Brandes, Stanley H. 1975. "Family Misfortune Stories in American Folklore." *Journal of the Folklore Institute* 12 (1):5–17.

Brandt, Allan M., and Paul Rozin, eds. 1997. *Morality and Health*. London: Routledge.

Broom, Dorothy, and Andrea Whittaker. 2004. "Controlling Diabetes, Controlling Diabetics: Moral Language in the Management of Diabetes Type 2." *Social Science & Medicine* 58:2371–82.

Browning, Frank. 2012. "Diabetes in Appalachia: 'Just give me a pill.'" *Salon* (August 8). http://www.salon.com/2012/08/08/diabetes_in_appalachia_just_give_me_a_pill.

Cattell-Gordon, David. 1990. "The Appalachian Inheritance: A Culturally-Transmitted Traumatic Stress Syndrome?" *Journal of Progressive Human Service* 1:41–57.

Collins, Patricia Hill. 2000. *Black Feminist Thought: Knowledge, Consciousness, and the Politics of Empowerment*. New York: Routledge.

Crawford, Robert. 1977. "You Are Dangerous to Your Health: The Ideology and Politics of Victim Blaming." *International Journal of Health Services* 7 (4):663–80.

———. 1980. "Healthism and the Medicalisation of Everyday Life." *International Journal of Health Services* 10:365–88.

Danielson, Larry. 1994. "Family Folklore Studies 1994." *Southern Folklore* 51:11–16.

Eisenman, David P., Kristina M. Cordasco, Steve Asch, Joya F. Golden, and Deborah Glik. 2007. "Disaster Planning and Risk Communication with Vulnerable Communities: Lessons from Hurricane Katrina." *American Journal of Public Health* 97 (S1):S109–S115.

Elder, Keith, Sudha Xirasagar, Nancy Miller, Shelly Ann Bowen, Saundra Glover, and Crystal Piper. 2007. "African Americans' Decisions Not to Evacuate New Orleans Before Hurricane Katrina: A Qualitative Study." *American Journal of Public Health* 97 (S1):S124–S129.

Family History Tool Project. 2005. *AFS Public Programs Bulletin* 22:6.

Goffman, Erving. 1963. *Stigma: Notes on the Management of Spoiled Identity*. New York: Simon and Schuster.

Goldstein, Diane, and Amy Shuman. 2012. "The Stigmatized Vernacular: Where Reflexivity Meets Untellability." *Journal of Folklore Research* 49 (2):113–26.

Goodwin, Joseph P. 1994. "My First Ex-Lover-In-Law: You Can Choose Your Family." *Southern Folklore* 51:35–47.

Hall, Sharon K. 2009. "Disasters and Psychological Risk in Children." In *Children, Law, and Disasters: What We Have Learned from Katrina and the Hurricanes of 2005*, 43–61. Houston: American Bar Association and the University of Houston.

Horigan, Kate Parker. 2013. "'They probably got us all on the news': Personal Narratives and Public Trauma in Post-Katrina New Orleans." PhD diss., Ohio State University.

Huckstep, Susan L. 2008. "The Media's Framing of Poverty Following Hurricane Katrina." PhD diss., Regent University.

Kotkin, Amy J., and Steven J. Zeitlin. 1983. "In the Family Tradition." In *Handbook of American Folklore*, ed. Richard M. Dorson, 90–99. Bloomington: Indiana University Press.

Lindahl, Carl. 2013. "Vernacular Self-Rescue: 'Victims' Save One Another and Themselves." In *Second Line Rescue*, ed. Barry Jean Ancelet, Marcia Gaudet, and Carl Lindahl. Jackson: University Press of Mississippi.

Lindenmeyer, Antje, Frances Griffiths, Eileen Green, Diane Thompson, and Maria Tsourou-fli. 2008. "Family Health Narratives: Midlife Women's Concepts of Vulnerability to Illness." *Health* 12 (3):275–93.

Link, Bruce G., and Jo C. Phelan. 2001. "Conceptualizing Stigma." *Annual Review of Sociology* 27:363–85.

Lupton, Deborah. 1995. *The Imperative of Health: Public Health and the Regulated Body*. London: Sage.

Morgan, Kathryn L. 1966. "Caddy Buffers: Legends of a Middle-Class Negro Family in Philadelphia." *Keystone Folklore Quarterly* 11:67–88.

———. 1980. *Children of Strangers: The Stories of a Black Family*. Philadelphia: Temple University Press.

Richards, Martin. 1997. "It Runs In the Family: Lay Knowledge about Inheritance." In *Culture, Kinship, and Genes: Towards Cross-Cultural Genetics*, ed. Angus Clarke and Evelyn Parsons, 175–94. New York: St. Martin's Press.

Rolland, John S. 1999. "Families and Genetic Fate: A Millenial Challenge." *Families Systems & Health* 17:123–32.

Scollan-Koliopoulos, Melissa. 2004. "Consideration for Legacies about Diabetes and Self-Care for the Family with a Multigenerational Occurrence of Type 2 Diabetes." *Nursing and Health Sciences* 6:223–27.

Thomas, Jeannie B. 1997. *Featherless Chickens, Laughing Women, and Serious Stories.* Charlottesville: University Press of Virginia.

Walter, F. M., and J. Emery. 2005. "'Coming Down the Line': Patients' Understanding of their Family History of Common Chronic Disease." *Annals of Family Medicine* 3 (5):405–14.

Walter, F. M., J. Emery, D. Braithwaite, and T. M. Marteau. 2004. "Lay Understanding of Familial Risk of Common Chronic Diseases: A Systematic Review and Synthesis of Qualitative Research." *Annals of Family Medicine* 2 (6):583–94.

Werner-Lin, Allison. 2007. "Danger Zones: Risk Perceptions of Young Women from Families with Hereditary Breast and Ovarian Cancer." *Family Process* 46:335–49.

Werner-Lin, Allison, and David S. Gardner. 2009. "Family Illness Narratives of Inherited Cancer Risk: Continuity and Transformation." *Families, Systems, & Health* 27 (3):201–12.

Wilson, William A. 1991. "Personal Narratives: The Family Novel." *Western Folklore* 50 (2):127–49.

Zeitlin, Steven J. 1980. "'An Alchemy of Mind': The Family Courtship Story." *Western Folklore* 39 (1):17–33.

Zeitlin, Steven J., Amy J. Kotkin, and Holly Cutting Baker. 1993. *A Celebration of American Family Folklore: Tales and Traditions from the Smithsonian Collection.* Cambridge, MA: Yellow Moon.

PART TWO

Folk Knowledge, Belief, and Treatment
in Regional and Ethnic Health Praxis

CHAPTER FOUR

Latina/o Local Knowledge about Diabetes: Emotional Triggers, Plant Treatments, and Food Symbolism

—Michael Owen Jones

Sitting on a well-worn sofa in the living room of her small apartment in Venice, California, the walls adorned with family photos and religious images, Silvia Herrera lists her relatives with diabetes.[1] They include her mother, an aunt, a nephew, and one brother—all of whom died of complications from the disease—along with another brother, two sisters, a grandson, and a six-year-old niece who are still living. Mrs. Herrera, an émigré from Guadalajara, has diabetes as well. The disorder has also beset Jorge Alvarez and his wife Rosa Alvarez, both from Jalisco, Mexico, who have had diabetes for thirty years and twenty years, respectively. Mr. Alvarez's father and grandfather suffered from diabetes, as did Mrs. Alvarez's father, two of her father's brothers, and two of her older sisters as well as her younger sister (who died at age sixty-five from the disease). None of Mr. and Mrs. Alvarez's three daughters has diabetes, but two of their four sons were diagnosed with the disease ten and eight years previously at ages thirty-nine and forty-two. A similar situation obtains for many other immigrants and Mexican Americans I have interviewed; they or a spouse or other family members have diabetes. Several have died from it.

Statistics released by the National Institute of Diabetes and Digestive and Kidney Diseases (NIDDK) for 2005, when I began my interviews, indicate that 23.9 percent of Latina/os aged forty-five to seventy-four are afflicted with diabetes compared to 12 percent of non-Hispanic whites. According to the NIDDK, 20.8 million people in the United States, or 7 percent of the population aged twenty or older, have this metabolic disorder, which is twice the proportion in 1993. Millions more have pre-diabetes consisting of impaired fasting glucose and impaired glucose tolerance. Diabetes is now the seventh leading cause of death in America.[2] The prevalence rate of adult-onset diabetes among African Americans, Latina/os, American Indians, and Native Hawaiians is two to three times that of non-Hispanic whites. These ethnic populations experience much higher rates of complications too, such as blindness, amputations, strokes, and heart disease, and twice as many as whites die from diabetes. Latina/os have a sixfold greater incidence of end-stage renal disease than do non-Hispanic whites, and they are much more likely to require insulin treatments, which many of them fear.

In this chapter, I discuss several areas of Latina/o local knowledge about diabetes.[3] First, I consider explanatory models regarding causes and the course of illness or disease, especially the role of emotional precipitants and aggravators of their condition. Second, I discuss the use of plants from cactus salad to horsetail tea and others in between in order to lower blood glucose levels, which seems to be effective. The third is awareness of non-nutritional meanings and uses of food—rituals, symbols, and sources of identity—that dieticians seem to seldom take into account but which render modifications in diet difficult. The fourth is self-reported "barriers" to maintaining a recommended dietary regimen, which go beyond several mentioned in the literature that tend to blame and stigmatize the patient. The fifth is perceptions of the social and psychological dimensions of illness that all too rarely are considered by medical personnel when treating diabetes among Latina/os.

My point is that systems of local knowledge regarding illness and healing, revealed through folkloristic ethnography, may be a source of insight for health education initiatives, the training of healthcare professionals, and developing and assessing intervention programs. In regard to the concept "local knowledge," I am following Vandebroek et al. (2011:1), who write that "Local Knowledge Systems (LKS) consist of the knowledge, beliefs, traditions, practices, institutions, and worldviews developed and sustained by indigenous and local communities, and [that] are believed to represent an adaptive strategy to the environment in which the communities live." Employing ethnography that involves in-depth interviews, observation, and other techniques to obtain qualitative data is particularly useful for discovering local knowledge and people's experiences such as reported here.

1. Causation and Exacerbation: The Role of Emotions and Stress

With no prompting other than my statement that I wanted to talk about diabetes, most of the twenty-eight individuals I interviewed in the Los Angeles area immediately launched into narratives about stressful life events that contributed to their disease, particularly in regard to causing or exacerbating it (see Appendix for a summary of information about interviewees). Martha Cruz, six months pregnant, came upon her husband's truck in the field, opened the door to greet him, and discovered to her horror that a corpse was behind the steering wheel. She collapsed from *susto* (fright). She was hospitalized with diabetes, her blood glucose so high that her unborn son's life was in danger. When I interviewed her in 2005, Mrs. Cruz was on hypoglycemic medications, insulin, and kidney dialysis. Breaking down in tears, she contended that she suffered a great setback in controlling her diabetes in 1993 when another son, washing his car in the alley in preparation of picking up his girlfriend, was shot and killed by a gang member.

"In my case," said Yolanda Lopez, "I believe it was *corajes* [fits of anger]. . . . I had a lot of problems with a neighbor and we were at each other's throats every day . . . and that was when it developed, I think . . . I believe that about this, it is more about one's character, one's problems, what one goes through. . . . I believe that there are some people that just 'swallow' everything. They have much mortification because of family problems and they become diabetics," a concept with which interviewees Josephina Rivera, José Lopez, and several others agreed.

Alicia Gutierrez has experienced a variety of strong emotions that precipitated or aggravated her diabetes beginning with *susto* and anger after she was stabbed by three youth attempting to steal her purse. Living alone since her husband's death in 2001, she suffers *tristeza* (deep sadness or depression) that has made her diabetes worse, she said, weeping as she tried to talk about it. Worry (*inquietude* or *preoccupado*) and anxiety (*nervios*) or an attack of severe anxiety (*ataque de nervios*) also can aggravate diabetes, which they have done in her case, she said. Even great joy (*gusto* or *alegria*) may trigger the disease, particularly when it is sudden and accompanied by such surprise as to be shocking.

Interviewees accepted to varying degrees biomedical hypotheses about the role of genetics, exercise, and diet. A few expressed uncertainty regarding the impact of diet on themselves or others, although many accepted it as a contributing factor, mentioning excessive consumption of sodas, pork, and starchy foods along with obesity and lack of exercise. Some suggested the possibility of toxins in the environment and food supply. No one said the illness was God's will, punishment for bad behavior, or fate. Most, however, referred to stressful events and extreme emotional states as precipitating the disorder in themselves or other people, or of making their condition worse. Thinking about the cause of her diabetes, Josephina Rivera said, "I carried a strong *coraje* [rage] . . . the most horrible thing in the world." According to Jorge Alvarez, "One time, well, for me I got really upset with someone, a woman and well, you know, you can't really let your steam off. . . . I couldn't relieve myself, because what can you tell a woman? When I got very mad, my legs used to hurt a lot and a little later I became ill with diabetes, I think, but that I am not sure." Similarly, Alicia Gutierrez commented, "I think sadness and getting mad [angry] and being scared." Yolanda Lopez also cited the power of emotions in combating the illness, noting that "*tristeza* [sadness] makes one not get out of bed and not eat right, of course. Yes, this also. There are many emotional aspects."

Attempting to comprehend their disease and why it had befallen them, several interviewees combined their understanding of a biomedical explanation—genetic susceptibility—with an intense and stressful emotional experience. Margarita Mendoza remarked, "I think because one already has the genes for it, any little thing that happens brings it on. . . . When one already has it through inheriting it, you have two things that work together and you end up developing it." As Adriana Moreno put it, "We all have diabetes in us; it just needs a trigger to bring it out." Yolanda Lopez implicated emotional triggers as "the most important thing, because my cousin's husband had a great *susto*. He is a thin man and that is how he developed his diabetes; he had had a terrible fright."

Ascribing the onset of diabetes to an intense emotional experience affords a reason why one person has the disease but other people who have eaten the same kinds and amount of food as that individual and exercised less do not have diabetes. Because Type 2 diabetes usually develops slowly over time as the pancreas is stressed, it is initially asymptomatic, and some of its physiological consequences might not seem connected to it. Identifying a sudden provoking factor may provide a sense of proximate cause of a condition that has existed for a while with no one's awareness of it.

Numerous works document Mexican Americans' reference to emotional triggers.[4] However, danger lies in the possibility of researchers treating the notion of emotional causes as simply a "cultural tradition."[5] Such a tendency is a form of essentializing that attributes patients' concepts and behaviors to little more than their ethnicity (Anderson, Blue, and Lau 1991). In contrast to this "cultural source hypothesis" is the "experiential source theory," which grants that many widely spread beliefs are supported by experiences that are reasonable, rationally developed from experience, and manifested "independently of a subject's prior beliefs, knowledge, or intention" (Hufford 1995:28). As David J. Hufford writes, some "beliefs show not only persistence but remarkable similarity from one tradition to another because they accurately recount observations which are themselves remarkably similar" (1995:31).

A growing body of literature concerning laboratory experiments with animals and human beings suggests that intensely felt emotions may indeed be linked to diabetes. Stress has long been suspected of having significant effects on metabolic activity. "Counter-regulatory" hormones appear to be released in response to stress, which results in elevated blood glucose levels and decreased insulin action (Surwit and Schneider 1993). Such an energy-mobilizing effect (the result of the fight or flight response) is beneficial (i.e., of adaptive importance) in a healthy organism. Stress-induced increases in blood glucose cannot be adequately metabolized, however, where there is a relative lack of insulin (Surwit and Williams 1996). In addition, psychological stress has been implicated as a link to psychoendocrinical pathways that cause insulin resistance (Schoenberg et al. 2005).

In national samples, depression appears two to three times greater among those with diabetes than in the general population (Brody et al. 2001; Hatcher and Whittemore 2007). Depression, however, is bi-directional (Vinicor and Jack 2004). It can cause decreased self-care, inadequate glycemic control, and diminished quality of life; in turn, interruptions in efforts to maintain behavioral changes may result in depression, anxiety, and diabetic anger that further impede efforts at self-maintenance regimens (Hall 1987).

Medical textbooks as well as publications from the NIDDK have ignored or minimized the salience of stress to diabetes. Nutrition education programs rarely include stress reduction or relaxation techniques but instead focus heavily on diet, exercise, adherence to testing blood glucose levels, and compliance with taking medications.[6] Some medical personnel and nutrition educators use scare tactics to promote adherence to prescribed behaviors by warning of severe complications of diabetes (amputations, blindness), undermining efforts to prevent or forestall these symptoms (Adams 2003; Schoenberg et al. 2005). Research on the role of stress in causing high blood glucose levels, making a patient's condition worse, interfering with efforts to manage the disease and its symptoms, and contributing to the development of complications, should be discussed in medical texts, included in the training of healthcare personnel, and incorporated into educational programs for the public.

2. Plant Treatments: From Cactus Salad to Horsetail Tea

The NIDDK insists that improved glycemic control through diet greatly benefits people with diabetes. The agency bemoans the fact that more than half of those known to have this disorder do not receive formal "self-control training." However, some Latina/os utilize certain plants to treat diabetes and the associated condition of hypertension, thereby exercising a degree of self-control by participating in the use of traditional remedies. In this section, I review some of the research on plant-based modalities and discuss uses of plant remedies by Mexicans and Mexican Americans whom I interviewed in Los Angeles.

The few surveys that have recorded information about herbal remedy use by Latina/os in the United States indicate that as many as 91 percent of the subjects in the studies have employed plant materials in treating diabetes.[7] In one research project, 84 percent of respondents cited herbs as possible alternative modalities whether they personally used them or not (Hunt, Arar, and Akana 2000). Among the small number of plants to treat diabetes that have been documented thus far from Latina/os in the United States are *nopal*, or prickly pear cactus (the most frequently mentioned plant in studies by Poss, Jezewski, and Stuart 2003; Coronado et al. 2004, and in my own research), along with *sábila* (aloe vera), *maguey* (century plant), *chaya* (vegetable pear), *barbas de elote* (corn silk), *lagrimas de San Pedro* (tears of St. Peter), *cola de caballo* (horsetail), *nispero* (loquat), *chaya* (vegetable pear), and *prodigiosa* (bricklebush).

"*Nopal*, it's good for diabetes and for other things," said Jorge Alvarez. "I try to give it to my wife by taking off the spines [on the pads] and then I toast it a bit on the skillet. I think this is the best way of eating the *nopal*." His wife, Rosa Alvarez, said, "I boil it to make a salad with onion and tomato." Mr. Alvarez also prepares a *licuado* or "smoothie" composed of raw items, which seems to be the common way of consuming cactus: *nopal* liquefied with *apio* (celery) and *berro* (watercress), along with a small amount of pineapple and apple juice (to reduce the sharp tang of the cactus), and ingested in the morning. Interviewees Josephina Rivera, Gabriela Diaz, and Margarita Mendoza also described *nopal* and other herbal beverages.

Most people I interviewed have gardens in which they grow a dozen or more plants having medicinal uses, along with other culinary plants and also those having dual purposes. Adriana Moreno has cultivated the area behind the apartment building where she lives in Venice, but in addition, she has "emergency plants" in hangers and pots on her balcony for times when one of her children wakes up in the middle of the night with an ailment, plants such as *borraja* (borage) to treat headaches or temperature, *hierba buena* (spearmint) and *estafiate* (artemisa or mugwort) for indigestion, *hierba santa* (blessed herb) for coughs, and *ruda* (rue) for ear infections.

A woman in City Terrace tends more than forty plants and a *curandero* (healer) in Echo Park has eighty.[8] Arturo Sandoval in Culver City grows about 150 plants in his front, side, and back yards, which includes some duplicates.

He remarked on the pleasure of digging the soil with his bare hands, the prettiness of the plants, including *nopal*, the sweetness of the fruit, and the beauty that the flowers and greenery contribute to his home. He is greatly appreciated for giving seasonal fruit as well as the flowers and leaves of medicinal plants to people at a senior center; several women combine the *cedron* (lemon verbena) and *cancerina* (Mexican heather) that he brings with *cuachalate* (a medicinal bark from Mexico), which they claim helps control their diabetes. Remarked Jorge Alvarez, "You can say that all plants have some medicinal purpose." Likewise, Gloria Aguilar affirmed, "I do believe in a lot of the healing properties of some of these plants." Identifying one as *hierba santa* [holy herb, blessed herb, or saint herb], Margarita Mendoza said, "To me all the herbs that are good are saints."

Many desert plants eaten as food or medicine, including *nopal*, aloe vera, and century plant, "contain mucilaginous polysaccharide gums that are viscous enough to slow the digestion and absorption of sugary foods" (Nabhan 1998:175). For instance, aloe gel contains glucomannan, a water-soluble fiber, and *nopal* "has a high-soluble fiber and pectin content, which may affect intestinal glucose uptake, partially accounting for its hypoglycemic actions" (Yeh et al. 2003:1286). There appears to be increased cellular sensitivity to insulin as well (Lopez 2007). Therefore, *nopal* and other desert plants likely reduce blood-sugar levels that stress the pancreas (which permanently damages insulin metabolism), or at least they prolong the period over which sugar is absorbed into the blood after one eats. Miguel Angel Gutierrez (1998) writes that possible ramifications "include diabetic patients reducing [the] dosage of current hypoglycemic agents by incorporating these plants into their diet. Also patients with mild Type 2 diabetes could possibly avoid the use of these agents and control blood glucose via diet alone."

Other frequently employed remedies for diabetes consist of teas. According to Silvia Herrera, one is made by boiling a handful of *matarique* (Indian plantain) leaves in a liter of water, which is drunk four or five times a day. Yolanda Lopez and Alicia Gutierrez mentioned *nispero* (loquat) tea using about three leaves per cup. Another remedy combines the leaves of *lagrimas de San Pedro* (tears of St. Peter) and the stems of *cola de caballo* (horsetail). "You get a little of each, a cup, like this, like four fingers per cup," explained Carlos Mendez. "You get the water first, boil it for five minutes and then you turn it off [and steep leaves in it]. [You drink it] in the morning and at night."

Several people I interviewed take such teas, which are diuretics, to lower blood glucose levels. A study of 31,512 adults found that treatment with a diuretic was not only less expensive but often more beneficial than a calcium channel blocker or an angiotensin-converting enzyme (ACE) inhibitor in protecting against stroke and heart attacks in people with diabetes and those with elevated fasting glucose (National Institute of Health 2005). Some interviewees were outspoken in their preference for herbal remedies over prescription drugs or advocated complementary rather than alternative use of them. Verónica Mendez summed up this attitude, saying, "If I could find something that's natural I would take it anytime more than the medications. The medications do you good for this, but then they harm you for that. Of course the natural herbs are a very slow process but they work."

Healthcare professionals tend to overlook or downplay the significance of folk and alternative medicine (Helton 1996; Jonas et al. 2013) rather than incorporate it into a plan of care (Davidhizar, Bechtel, and Giger 1998). Several authors of works about diabetes among Latina/os consider traditional therapies to be "negative health practices" (Brown et al. 2002), "noncongruent cultural beliefs" (Philis-Tsimikas et al. 2004), and potentially dangerous owing to the chance of people using them for the wrong indications and possible interactions with prescription medications (Poss, Jezewski, and Stuart 2003:319) or because of the toxicity of certain plants as well as the prospect of perhaps triggering a hypoglycemic crisis when herbal remedies are combined with oral therapies or insulin (Tripp-Reimer et al. 2001).

A detailed review of clinical trials of herbs employed in treating diabetes, however, found that *nopal* and aloe vera showed positive results as hypoglycemic agents and, further, that there were no apparent side effects (Yeh et al. 2003).[9] Some contend that the use of herbs will result in people not taking their prescribed medications or monitoring their blood sugar levels (Pegado, Kwan, and Medeiros 2003). On the other hand, in a community in Mexico, "better diabetes control was related to a higher level of cultural knowledge," that is, awareness and use of traditional modalities (Daniulaityte 2004:1889), and in a group of Mexican Americans in South Texas "those patients very actively using alternative approaches also tended to be very actively using biomedical methods; they were using all resources they encountered" (Hunt, Arar, and Akana 2000:216). As Verónica Mendez said, "Yeah, if you want to get cured you try anything they tell you, you know?"

Few of the interviewees told medical personnel about their ideas of the emotional causes of diabetes or about their using plants as hypoglycemic agents. "They don't believe in them," stated Margarita Mendoza. Most of the ones who did tell doctors about their conceptions and plant treatments were ignored or even chastised (as noted also by Shelley et al. 2009). "Have you ever told your doctor about the *nopal*, that you take it?," I asked Josephina Rivera. "No," she replied. "Why not?" As she explained, "There's no point, they don't believe in that. They don't listen. Why should one tell them? One just takes it and if it does one good then it's good, and if it does one bad." I asked Jorge Alvarez, too, about his interaction with medical personnel, specifically if he had told his doctor about using *lagrimas de San Pedro* and *cola de caballo*. "Yeah. He is not happy with it." I also mentioned the cactus, to which Mr. Alvarez replied that the doctor told him, "I know you take it but I am not happy about that."

In concluding this section, I would note that laboratory studies strongly suggest that several plants appear efficacious as well as safe in treating diabetes and associated diseases. As the authors of one review of 108 trials involving 36 herbs and 9 supplements write, medical personnel should "keep an open mind in advising patients who might already be using these" treatments (Yeh et al. 2003:1289). Further, "They should be guided not only by sound clinical judgment, but also by patients' preferences, needs, and values" (1290). *Nopal*, aloe vera, and other plants are familiar to people who know of their use traditionally in their families and communities. Some individuals prefer "natural medicine" to prescription drugs. Those who cultivate medicinal herbs in their yards appear to derive sensory and aesthetic pleasure from looking at the plants and breaking off a leaf, crushing it, and smelling the aroma as well as making teas and tinctures with them. For everyone I interviewed, growing and utilizing medicinal plants symbolizes self-reliance. When standard interventions fail, incorporating phytomedicine with proven hypoglycemic effects in the treatment plan might prove attractive and effective.

Ritual, Symbol, and Sacrifice: Non-Nutritional Meanings of Food

Non-nutritional meanings and uses of food is a third area about which qualitative research can uncover local knowledge. "Food is never just something to eat," writes Margaret Visser in *Much Depends on Dinner* (1986:14). "Desserts: those are my comfort foods," declared Gloria Aguilar. "I do crave my little chocolate," said Elizabeth Castillo. Individuals convey feelings toward others through offerings of food; rejecting the food may be construed as a rejection of the host. Remarked Gabriela Diaz: "I feel bad when I refuse to eat food that friends offer me. I don't like to explain my health to everybody so I say no thank you, and they say, 'Why don't you like this?'" When Yolanda Lopez goes to someone's home, she admitted "I eat as if I am not diabetic." Rita Valdez said that most people know she is diabetic but they nevertheless insist that she eat the foods they have prepared, "so I take only a small bite."

Impacting the choice of fare is that food is gendered. Typically meat and starches are masculine, while chicken, fish, and fruit are feminine, which strongly affects efforts to modify men's diets (Heisley 1990; Jones 2007; Sobal 2005). Also affecting food choice is the conception of a "proper" meal (Douglas 1972; Kerr and Charles 1986) and the notion of a "complete" meal (Schlundt, Hargreaves, and Buchowski 2003), whether this includes dessert or some other item: "Many people feel if rice isn't cooked [and served], they haven't eaten," observed one woman (quoted in Beoku-Betts 1995:543). Food often conjures up fond memories: "I know that some of our traditional foods are not full of nutrients but they bring back good memories of childhood and I'm not giving them up just because some researcher says they are bad" (quoted in James 2004:358). Food defines events, whether a holiday, a family reunion, or a picnic at the beach. Food *is* the event in the case of many Latina/o families and communities joining together to make tamales during the Christmas season (Brown et al. 1981).

The preparation, service, and consumption of food, then, are fraught with meanings and meaningfulness and serve as a basis for meaning-making. Not surprisingly, food is also inextricably bound up with self and self-making, from family, regional, and ethnic identity to personal characteristics (Jones 2007). "Yes, I like to cook. And unfortunately, I like *what* I cook!," said Margarita Mendoza. Remarked Elizabeth Castillo: "I am a bread-eater; I am a sweet-eater. I'm sure that I'm like an alcoholic but with regard to sweets." Yolanda Lopez contended that since developing diabetes, "My life has changed a lot. You aren't able to eat whatever you want or what you like." Verónica Mendez also conceded the impact of diabetes on her eating habits: "It's affected me a lot 'cause I love my tortillas. I don't eat as many vegetables or salads as I would like to because I don't love my salads. . . . I need my beans and my tortillas. I have two friends . . . they were borderline diabetic . . . one of them lost so much weight . . . both of them did it. But they really sacrificed a lot and I said, I don't know. . . . I can sacrifice, but not as much as they did."

As Mrs. Mendez's remark indicates, "sacrifice" means to suffer loss, to give up something cherished, to renounce or surrender for an ideal, a belief, or an end. A number of interviewees bemoaned having to give up rice and beans and other items common to many Latina/os' diets as well as foods specific to the holiday season and being unable to eat what they liked or what was served at family get-togethers (see also Hatcher and Whittemore 2007; von Goeler et al. 2003). In a study by Carmen Rivera Adams (2007), one person said to the researcher: "We Puerto Ricans love our *pasteles* [meat pies], rice, beans, chicken, other meats. But, look, the diabetic can't eat any of that" (261). Clearly, clinicians need to pay attention to language in counseling. The use of negative terms such as *give up, do without,* and *cannot eat* may result in feelings of failure and low self-esteem among patients unable to achieve the ideal. This is apparent in metaphors employed by a patient suggesting that he or she is a naughty child, a foolish adult, or beyond redemption. "I mean, it's just ... we're bad ... we are," said Elizabeth Castillo who, with her husband, has struggled often unsuccessfully to control diabetes through diet. "We're just bad, period."

Why people think they must sacrifice foods they have known since child-hood, identify with, and prefer owing to its flavoring as a distinctive marker of cuisine (Rozin 1982) has not been explained. Scarcely any cookbooks exist for Latina/os with diabetes, and recipes in educational materials usually describe American-style foods and eating habits. Although the California State Health Department's "5 a Day" nutritional guide contains scores of recipes, unfortunately it includes only two dips, one side dish, and an entrée as "Mexican" (a pan-ethnic label used by whites that offends many Central Americans in the state). In regard to *Comer Bien Para Vivir Mejor* (Eat Well to Live Better), a booklet distributed some years ago by the California Diabetes Control Pro-gram, Teri A. Hall (1987:283) writes, "Fortunately, traditional Mexican foods such as beans, rice, and tortillas lend themselves easily to the high-fiber, low-fat diet recommended for management of diabetes. The *Comer Bien* plan," which she helped to develop, "instead of prescribing an unfamiliar eating pat-tern, illustrates ways to modify methods of preparation of traditional foods (e.g., using less oil or lard, grilling instead of frying)." In addition, "Menus for the high-fiber, low-fat food plan make daily use of beans and tortillas, with frequent use of rice, Mexican cheese (*queso fresco*), avocadoes, tomatoes, and cereals" as well as *nopal*, used also as a hypoglycemic agent.

Other interventions, however, usually consist of "knowledge transfer" that conveys information to patients about diabetes and its treatment along with "skills acquisition" in taking medications and reading glucose levels. Predictably, assessing the success of programs entails determining adherence behaviors and measuring such physiologic outcomes as levels of weight, fit-ness, cholesterol, and blood glucose. The prevailing paradigm in nutrition research and interventions boils down to a technological model, one preoc-cupied with intakes and outputs, and with weights, levels, scores, scales, and other measurable results (Sharman et al. 1991:261). Most interventions are intensive, short-term efforts aimed at achieving quantifiable objectives. Virtu-ally all programs of nutritional education and behavioral change are claimed to be effective; within the assumptive framework employed, they probably do show improvements in technical areas of skills, knowledge, and monitor-ing. In addition, the Hawthorne effect is likely at work, that is, the activities of people who know they are being observed tend to conform to what the experimenters expect of them.[10]

A few researchers have censured the assumption that knowledge transfer is a panacea for changing behavior and maintaining alterations in lifestyle after program completion (Campbell et al. 1996; Liburd 2003; Rubin, Peyrot, and Saudek 1991). According to a literature review by Glazier et al. (2006), "Interventions that were consistently associated with the largest negative outcomes included those that used mainly didactic teaching or that focused only on diabetes knowledge" (1675). In one study, twenty-four of thirty participants had seen a nutritionist but few returned because "The dietary advice they received did not take their cultural traditions into consideration" (von Goeler et al. 2003:667). Other researchers contend that many projects directed at the poor involve norms decreed by those with power (Counihan 1999:123), are class-based and ethnocentric, and pathologize the tastes of others who lack the right cultural knowledge to eat "properly" (Ashley et al. 2004:61). Diabetics identifying themselves as ethnic minorities charge that nutritional information is not specific to their own traditions or in a language comprehensible to them, that publications are bereft of images of people like themselves, and that the recipes "are for things I would never eat" (quoted in James 2004:359). The issues of living and coping with diabetes suggest the need to shift from a knowledge model to patient-centered perspectives, self-management, and empowerment (Glasgow and Osteen 1992).

To maximize the good that they do, clinicians should understand the impact of customs and symbolism on identity and food choice. One way to achieve this goal might be to draw upon a list of general questions to obtain information from patients.[11] Devising a list of questions is not a recipe for success, however. Clinicians' perspectives need to change from strict adherence to technological and compliance models to approaches that emphasize collaboration, negotiation, and the joint development of treatment plans that the patient can live with, plans that are appropriate to the symbolic significance of food in the patient's daily life, social relations, and self-making. To gain this orientation, healthcare personnel should identify assumptions in their own system of beliefs, for example, that patients who do not practice healthful behaviors do not care about their well-being, that biomedicine is "right," that traditional beliefs must be changed rather than built upon, that people should and will follow instructions given by health practitioners, and that adherence failure is the patient's fault and problem (Tripp-Reimer 2001). They can also reflect on their own symbolic uses of food socially and emotionally, which may generate greater understanding of and empathy toward patients.[12] As Bisogni et al. (2002) assert, "Learning about the identities that clients bring to and derive from eating can help practitioners to think about food through the eyes of their clients and forces practitioners to see beyond their own personal or professional meanings for food and eating" (137).

Barriers to Diet and Exercise: Who, or What, Is to Blame?

A fourth topic is that of the challenges faced by diabetics in attempting the self-management of their condition as articulated by the patients themselves. Researchers have hypothesized a long list of barriers.[13] One set consists of *patient factors*, such as poor knowledge about diabetes, low literacy, limited preventive attitude, low socioeconomic status, deficient English language skills, low acculturation levels, and poor motivation to control their condition. Another is *provider factors* like clinician-patient communication in need of improvement. A third is comprised of *system factors* including overstressed physicians, insufficient incentives to healthcare personnel, and imperfect organizational models. Yet another is *structural or environmental barriers* such as unavailable physical resources, including transportation; neighborhood grocery stores selling affordable, healthful food; and exercise facilities. Reference to patient factors has a negative tone and often involves victim blaming and stigmatizing (Broom and Whittaker 2004; Oomen, Owen, and Suggs 1999).

Interviewees identify stressors other than those mentioned above. Self-reported difficulties include being forced to follow a prescribed diet that does not involve traditional foods and customary flavors. "I cannot eat good if I don't have my salsa in my food all the time," insisted Gabriela Diaz. I asked Rita Valdez what was the most difficult to refrain from eating. "Tortillas!" She avoids flour tortillas now but at each meal eats one made of corn. She particularly misses, and often craves, enchiladas, *chili rellenos*, *pozole*, and *menudo*. Holidays and family get-togethers are especially problematic. Josephina Rivera said, "The day of Thanksgiving . . . that one pie made of pumpkin: I know that I shouldn't eat it, but I get tempted and I take nibbles . . . nibbles." Remarked Margarita Mendoza, "It's just that sometimes when there's a gathering or a party I eat the sweets that are there. I can't help myself and I have them. I don't stick strictly to my diet." And although Martha Cruz is on five oral medications, insulin, and dialysis, she also cannot entirely forego special dishes at parties and festive occasions.

To the consternation of some family members, others are in denial about their condition; no matter the concern expressed or assistance offered, the diabetic person refuses to address the situation. Many individuals with diabetes crave foods they have been told not to eat such as sweets, pork, enchiladas, cheese-filled chilies, fried meats, and flour tortillas (or corn tortillas made with lard in the *masa* [dough made of corn], which renders the dough smooth). Said Yolanda Lopez, "I really like *dulce de leche* [milk candy] but I can't eat it. I only have small bites. I only eat chocolate every once in a while and I really like it." Elizabeth Castillo admitted that "What's difficult for me is to give up desserts, and chocolate desserts in particular; it's very difficult for me to say, 'Oh, no thank you.'" "But those are my comfort foods," added her sister Gloria Aguilar.

Another concern is not being counseled in how to deal with the emotional, social, and symbolic aspects of food (Adams 2003; Jones 2007). Then there is the high cost of healthful foods and their absence in certain areas of the city. Not having instruction in how to modify less healthful preparations of foods also confounds efforts at pursuing dietary changes. Another problem is the fact that restaurants and fast food chains offer few if any dishes that people with diabetes can eat (Adams 2003), and many still do not label menu items with their content or calorie count (Diamant et al. 2007). The lack of healthful foods in the workplace creates problems for some (Jack 2004). In addition, a patient, particularly a woman, may view dietary changes as "selfish or a burden to her family as well as costly and insignificant to the family's overall well-being" (Oomen, Owen, and Suggs 1999:222).

Feeling bored, hungry, or dissatisfied with an often bland and sometimes expensive diet is not unusual.[14] Francisca Perez, whose husband, Juan Perez, is on dialysis, told me that she found it too difficult to make different preparations for family members three times a day, so she purchased food for her husband from a home-delivery service that was recommended to her:

> He said, "What kind of diet is this?" The meat, he didn't like the meat. It's true that they didn't put salt on it, but sometimes they put this gravy on and he didn't like it. He stayed with it for a month. For a month [weekdays only, not weekends] we paid $1,000. . . . And he wasn't happy. He said, "No, I don't like this food." And so, from the last foods they brought, I threw away about five plates of already made food. It wasn't fresh. They would bring it, and then I would have to refrigerate it and then heat it up in the microwave. And the last foods he didn't want anymore. . . . I threw them away! And it came to about $15 per plate.

All of the issues mentioned in the preceding two paragraphs revolve around food. Another concern, however, is financial; not only the cost of food but also of prescription drugs. Half a dozen oral medications are prescribed by physicians to treat individuals with diabetes. These include drugs to stimulate the pancreas to produce more insulin, help the pancreas deliver insulin more quickly, make a person more sensitive to insulin, decrease the amount of glucose made by the liver, and slow the absorption of starches that one eats. Nearly all those with diabetes whom I interviewed rely on medications for other ailments as well. Juan Perez swallows fifteen different pills a day for hypertension, high cholesterol, diabetes, and other health problems. Josephina Rivera takes four medications, one of which has caused swelling in her legs. Margarita Mendoza is on ten medications, several of which produce unwanted side effects such as a constant dry cough. Roberto Herrera said, "I take a lot of pills for the prostate, for cholesterol, for diabetes, for . . . but in the long run everything does harm, I think. The plants are better."

Many of the people I interviewed are retired; a number have annual incomes of $10,000 or less for the household. The cost of medications overwhelms some budgets; for instance, Alicia Gutierrez spends $350 per month for them out of her income of $780. Among other health problems, Rafael Mendoza, a retired billing clerk for a trucking company, has a heart condition and his wife, Margarita Mendoza, who had worked in a beauty salon, has diabetes. They live in an apartment. Their annual income is less than $20,000 combined. Medications for each cost about $400 a month for a total of $800. How can they afford it? "We just cut our prescriptions in half. The pills, we just cut them in half. That's the only way." Like a number of others, they take a bus periodically from a local senior center to Tijuana where they purchase their medications at half the price charged by pharmacies in the United States.

Yet another hindrance to seeking help for diabetes is the attitude and behavior of some clinicians. Patients remark on the lack of communication, being rebuked for their traditional ideas and practices, suffering long waits at the office or clinic, and being given short shrift by personnel. "Do you know what caused your diabetes?," I asked Rosa Alvarez. "No." Her husband Jorge added, "The doctors never tell us." Alicia Gutierrez complained that doctors do not take time to listen to or discuss matters with older sick people like her. "They just take tests but they don't tell me why." Francisca Perez was concerned that at least one of her husband's medications caused diarrhea, "but the doctors don't ask or care." Josephina Rivera wonders if there is a possibility of an interaction between her medications and the *nopal* she uses, but she feels she cannot ask because clinicians will not listen to her. "The doctors don't tell me anything," complained Margarita Mendoza. "I have a doctor who . . . it's not right to speak of the doctors but . . . she doesn't let me get a word in. She says, 'I don't have time! I don't have time!' She just writes down what the nurse wrote down [the prescriptions] I was low on and she leaves. She doesn't give a chance to talk." Rafael Mendoza added: "We're going to change doctors.

There's another one here in Fox Hills." "But most of the doctors are like this," Mrs. Mendoza contended. Her husband has "had to get mad with the doctors in order for them to listen to us." Additionally, Mr. Mendoza argued: "Because money is there, they're curing money, not patients. They have too many patients. . . . They can't do anything. The doctor doesn't listen. I have been many years suffering from pain in my thigh. I want to explain that on certain days it hurts tremendously, but she says I'm telling her too much and that she doesn't have time until next time."

As Martínez and Carter-Pokras (2006) discovered through interviews with diabetes patients, "Promptness and politeness were important in determining good service" (903). Many of the providers in their study expressed a desire to build trusting relationships with Latina/o patients, understand their health beliefs and healing practices, and learn about community resources and support networks. Greene and Yedidia (2005) note that "Diabetes patients with highly positive assessments of their provider's support engage in self-management tasks approximately one day more often per week than those who hold negative views" (816). Despite the benefits to patients of a satisfactory relationship with clinicians, a long list of obstacles stand in patients' way of gaining information and services, communication between providers and patients is often flawed, and health disparities continue.

Conclusion: Social and Psychological Dimensions of Diabetes, and the Need for New Models, Programs, and Practices

The social and psychological dimensions of illness loom large in regard to diabetes as evident in people's narratives. "In daily life, Hispanic adults reported that diabetes affected the way they felt, how others perceived them, and their role in society," write Hatcher and Whittemore (2007:539); moreover, "several Hispanic adults felt as if having diabetes had become their whole identity and separated them from others." The disease affects the family as well. There is the burden of preparing different meals or the challenge of changing family members' tastes to accommodate the diet of the diabetic. Sometimes traditional roles are reversed, with children admonishing adults to check their blood pressure and telling them what they should or should not eat. Diabetes impacts the patient's social life, from having to explain his or her condition to being reproached about food selections by well-meaning friends and family, to having to reject food offered by others, food that often is considered the quintessential expression of friendship, love, and hospitality.

For their own good, people are urged to alter long-standing eating habits that involve sensory experiences, extranutritional meanings, and symbolic uses of food. Many find this is exceedingly difficult. Remarked Josephina Rivera: "There are times I see ice cream [sold by vendors] in the streets and my mouth waters, and I say, 'Oh, my God!' I tell my daughters that one day, when I know I am really sick, I am going to eat a really big one, even if I die—but I will die happy. The day will arrive, but not yet. . . . One makes a huge sacrifice. A lot of sacrifice."

Living with diabetes imposes great demands on patients who must test their blood sugar level several times a day, plan meals that balance food group selections, calculate calories and fat content, schedule exercise in relation to eating, and in advanced stages of the disease take medications orally or by injection daily. Local knowledge reveals that diabetes is not only pathophysiological; it is also social, cultural, and psychological. Both clinical practice and public health need to be more fully oriented to these aspects of the disease. In recent years, a number of articles about ethnic beliefs and practices conclude by calling for culturally sensitive, culturally appropriate, culturally competent, and culturally relevant health care (Whittemore 2008). A seeming paradox at first, what we appear to be dealing with is not necessarily cultural and not reducible to a patient's ethnicity, but more likely universal experiences and concerns in the human condition. Documents and programs originating with national and state agencies should counsel people in regard to emotional stress, the impact on the family, and the effect on social relations. Training for physicians, nurses, and nutritionists should contain information that includes people's use of herbal treatments, the non-nutritional meanings and uses of food, and the psychological and social aspects of diabetes in order for clinicians to better communicate with, guide, and help their patients. Otherwise, those with diabetes will not be adequately equipped to deal with their illness, forestall or prevent complications, and maximize their quality of life.

Appendix: Table of Sociodemographics, Cause of Diabetes, and Plant Treatments

Nearly all interviewees discussed the triggers or aggravators of diabetes using Spanish terms, which I reproduce here. The emotions and their English translations are, in alphabetical order: *coraje* (rage or intense anger), *gusto* (joy; or *alegria*, great joy), *inquietude* (worry; or *preoccupado*, worry), *nervios* (nerves; or *un ataque de nervios*, anxiety attack), *susto* (fright), and *tristeza* (sadness or depression).

Table 4.1								
Name	DOB	Where Born, and How Identify Self	When Migrate	Education	Income/Job	Diabetes in Self and/or Family	Emotions as Triggers or Aggravators	Plants Used for Diabetes
Aguilar, Gloria	1933	US; American and Latina	n/a	16 years	Nurse; $40,000–$50,000	Self, older sister (Elizabeth Castillo), brother (for 22 years)	Possibly susto as cause for others	Wants to try nopal
Alvarez, Jorge	1928	Tepatitlan, Jalisco, Mex.; Mexican	1956	6 years	Retired shoe maker, then cook; $12,000	Self (for 30 years), father, grandfather, 2 of their 4 sons (at ages 42 and 39)	Coraje as cause in self	Nopal; lagrimas de San Pedro and cola de caballo combined
Alvarez, Rosa	1932	Mexico; Mexican	1964	6 years	See husband Jorge	Self (for 20 years), father, 2 paternal uncles, brother (for 15 years), 2 of their 4 sons (at ages 42 and 39)	Tristeza and coraje as cause in self; nervios as aggravator	None mentione
Castillo, Elizabeth	1936	US; American and Latina	n/a	14 years	Retired sales rep.; more than $50,000 with husband	Self (for 10 years), younger sister (Gloria Aguilar), brother (for 22 years); one daughter	None for family; possibly coraje for other people	Wants to try herbs
Cruz, Martha	1953	Aquascalientes, Central Mexico	?	7 years	See husband Miguel	Self (for 21 years), mother	Susto as cause for self; coraje and tristeza as aggravators	Herbs not seemed to work (is on 5 oral medications, insulin, and dialysis 3 times per week)
Cruz, Miquel	1944	Nayarit, western Mexico	1981	1 year	Factory worker soon to retire; $14,000	Older sister, 3 younger brothers	Probably susto and coraje as cause for siblings	
Diaz, Gabriela	1922	Mazatlan, Sinaloa, Mexico; Mexican	1949	12 years	Worked in med supply co.; husband (now dead) worked on airplanes; $10,236 (she cares for 90-year old father at home)	Self (for 4 years), mother (at age 50)	Inquietude as cause for her	None mentione
Garcia, Ana María	1932	US; Mexican American	n/a	0 years	Worked for Pac Bell, receives Social Security; see husband Manuel	2 brothers (1 died in his late 50s), 2 sisters, 3 nephews (2 died of it), 1 grandson, 1 niece (age 6)	Susto and inquietude as causes; tristeza as aggravator	Nopal and loquat as preventatives
Garcia, Manuel	1932	US, Mexican American	n/a	10 years	Laborer for city; $20,000 combined with wife	Self; 2 cousins on father's side	None	None (afraid of drug interaction

ame	DOB	Where Born, and How Identify Self	When Migrate	Education	Income/Job	Diabetes in Self and/or Family	Emotions as Triggers or Aggravators	Plants Used for Diabetes
errera, berto	1937	Torrion, Guadalajara; Mexican	2003	6 years	Worked in water heater factory, now retired; less than $10,000	Cousins; not have diabetes himself but takes herbals as preventative		Matarique, nopal smoothies with sábila; prodigiosa and ajenjo teas when angry
errera, via	1941	Guadalajara; Mexican	2002	6 years	See husband Roberto	Self, sister	Inquietude as cause for her	Matari-que, nopal smoothies with sábila
pez, José	1932	Pegueros, Mexico; Mexican American	1961		Gardener; $30,000-$40,000	Wife; granddaughter		
pez, landa	1933	Jalisco, Mexico; Mexican American	1963		See husband José	Self (for 7 years); granddaughter	Coraje as cause for self	Berro, Florsensé (commercial preparation), discontinued nispero leaf tea because of acid stomach
endez, rlos		1940	Jalisco, Mexico	1956	5 years	Part-time gardener and retired machinist; $18,000	Self	Nispero leaf tea; lagrimas de San Pedro and cola de caballo combined
endez, rónica	1942	US; Mexican American	n/a	10 years	Makes and sells 70-80 tamales per week for $1 each; combined with husband's retirement	Self (for 3 years), sister (died 2005 at age 65), younger brother, mother, cousin, nephew (age 34)	Coraje as cause for self; other emotions aggravate her condition	Tried chaya leaves, loquat, lagrimas de San Pedro, and Milagrosa (commercial tea) but suffered acid stomach so ceased using it
endoza, argarita	1938	Mexico City; Mexican American	1970	10 years	Worked in beauty salon; see husband Rafael	Self (for 25 years), father (at age 65), mother (at age 40), cousin (at age 29 who died of it at age 35), son (for 6 years)		Nopal, pasto grama, hojas de aquacate tea, nispero leaf tea
endoza, fael	1940	California; Mexican American	n/a	9 years	Retired billing clerk for trucking co.; $10,000-$20,000 combined with wife;	Wife; son (for 6 years)		
preno, driana	1961	Aquascalientes, Central Mexico	?	7 years	Husband a maintenance man at convalescent hospital; $20,000-$30,000 (supports family of 5	Sister, mother	Susto as cause for sister	Prodigiosa tea when angry as preventative

Name	DOB	Where Born, and How Identify Self	When Migrate	Education	Income/Job	Diabetes in Self and/or Family	Emotions as Triggers or Aggravators	Plants Used for Diabetes
Perez, Juan	1923	Hanford CA; Mexican American	n/a	6 years	Retired Boeing gardener; $20,000 (supports 3 in family)	Self (for 30 years), younger brother, mother (at age 65)		None (is on 15 medications daily as well as dialysis 3 times per week)
Ramirez, Alejandra	1933	Jalisco, Mexico; Mexican	?	12 years	Retired teacher's aide; social security; see husband Pedro Ramirez	Self (for 2 years), younger sister (at age 45; now dead), older sister, younger brother	Inquietude as cause for self; coraje as cause for younger sister; tristeza as cause for older sister; coraje and inquietude as aggravators for brother	Nopal (also drinks parsley pancreas)
Ramirez, Pedro	Jalisco, Mexico; Mexican	?	0 years	Gardener; $10,000-$20,000 combined with wife	1 brother, 1 sister			
Rivera, Josepina	1924	Mexico City; Mexican	1980	2 years	Late husband in military; less than $10,000	Self, daughter (for 2 years), mother's sister	Coraje as cause; tristeza as aggravator	Nopal
MM-4(f) Ruiz, Teresa	1946	Los Angeles, CA; American	n/a	14 years	Hairdresser and owner of novelty store, husband a barber; $40,000-$50,000 combined (supports 3 in family)	Father, mother, sister, older brother, grandmother, grandfather	Does not believe	Mother used nopal smooth; also matarique
EC(m) Sandoval, Arturo	1931	Texas; Mexican American	n/a	2 years	Retired house painter; $13,000 (daughters pay mortgage utilities, some food)	2 brothers (died of it at ages 55 and 65), 1 sister (died of it at age 55), mother (died of it at age 77)	Possibly susto or coraje can be a cause for other people	Sábila tea as preventative
OM(F) Valdez, Rita	1936	Jalisco, Mexico; Mexicana	1972	7 years	Retired nanny; less than $10,000 (supports 3 in the family)	Self (for 20 years)	Susto and inquietude as cause; tristeza and coraje as aggravators	Nopal smooth
MN(f) Vargas, María	1922	Mazatlán, Mexico; Mexican	1949	12 years	Retired factory worker; $10,000	Self (for 3 years)	Tristeza as cause for her	None (afraid of effects)

Most interviewees mentioned the Spanish names for herbs utilized in the treatment of diabetes, which I cite here along with their English common names. In alphabetical order, they are *ajenjo* (wormwood, mugwort), *berro* (watercress), *chaya* (vegetable pear), *cola de caballo* (horse tail), *hojas de aquacate* (avocado leaves), *lagrimas de San Pedro* (Job's Tears), *matarique* (Indian plantain), *nispero* (loquat), *nopal* (prickly pear cactus), *pasto grama* (Blue Grama grass), *prodigiosa* (bricklebush), and *sábila* (aloe).

Notes

1. Pseudonyms for interviewees are used throughout this essay.

2. This 2011 figure was reported by the Center for Disease Control. http://www.cdc.gov/Diabetes/pubs/estimates11.htm (accessed March 21, 2014).

3. This research project was funded by a grant from the UCLA Center on Research, Education, Training and Strategic Communications on Minority Health Disparities, which is directed by Dr. Vickie Mays, and by a faculty research grant from the UCLA Committee on Research (COR). The study received approval from UCLA's Institutional Review Board in July 2005. I thank my former graduate student, Ms. Mary Helen de la Peña Brown (master's thesis, Folklore and Mythology, UCLA), for her help with the project.

The study involved convenience sampling. Most interviewees lived in Venice, California, but a few resided in adjacent Santa Monica and Culver City. They were known to my assistant Mary Helen de la Peña Brown from her thirty years of teaching in elementary schools in the area and her time on the Los Angeles City Council. Interviews were undertaken in respondents' homes; usually, husbands and wives were interviewed together. Most interviews were conducted in Spanish, but a few were in English and others in a mixture of the two. All were videotaped, transcribed, and translated into English. Photographs were taken of yards where respondents grew plants for medicinal purposes.

The project employed semi-structured interviews. After being given information regarding the study, the twenty-eight respondents were asked about the nature and causes of diabetes, which included biomedical explanations as well as emotional triggers and aggravators (along with how and why a strong emotion precipitates or exacerbates diabetes). Interviewees were queried about who in the family has diabetes and how long ago it developed. They were asked about using plants to treat their diabetes and their communication with healthcare personnel concerning their ideas about the causes and herbal treatments of this metabolic disorder. They were asked about their management of the disease, which comprised such topics as food choices and habits (as well as cravings), barriers to and motivations for seeking clinicians' help in maintaining a prescribed diet, and how having diabetes affected not only their identity and activities but also relationships with family and friends. Finally, sociodemographic information was solicited: date of birth, birthplace and how they identified themselves, when they immigrated, years of schooling, and annual income (in $10,000 increments beginning with $0–10,000, although several people indicated specific amounts). Pseudonyms are used throughout this essay, randomly selected from among common names of people of Mexican descent.

Nobody stated or implied a lack of health insurance, whether Medi-Cal, Medicare, and/or some form of Blue Cross. All diabetes patients had had medications prescribed for them (often several drugs were prescribed because of multiple chronic diseases), which, however, were not covered fully by insurance. The principal question asked of those on medications was not which drugs but which plants were utilized. With the exception of Gabriela Diaz, who occasionally stopped taking prescription drugs to cut costs, and Carlos Mendez, whose blood sugar levels were under control, no one relied on herbs exclusively.

4. See, for example, Arcury et al. (2004); Caban and Walker (2006); Coronado, Thompson, Tejeda et al. (2004); Daniulaityte (2004); Hunt, Valenzuela, and Pugh (1997; 1998); Hunt, Arar, and Akana (2000); Jezewski and Poss (2002); Poss and Jezewski (2002); and Weller et al. (1999).

5. Representatives of different ethnic groups, not just Latina/os, contend that intense emotions precipitate diabetes. For instance, Mull, Nguyen, and Mull (2001) elicited strong emotions (especially worry and sadness) from Vietnamese refugees in Orange County, California, as a cause of their metabolic disorder. Many of the British Bangladeshis interviewed by Greenhalgh, Helman, and Chowdhury (1998) mentioned physical or psychological stress. According to the literature reviewed by Rock (2003), Native Americans often claim distress and duress as the etiology of their disease. Two other studies involving multiple ethnic populations composed of African Americans, Latina/os, and whites (Loewe and Freeman 2000) and of African Americans, Mexican Americans, Great Lakes Indians, and whites (Schoenberg et al. 2005) report stressful events as a major factor in diabetes etiology, according to interviewees.

6. For a critique of the compliance model, see Anderson and Funnell (2000).

7. Reported percentages vary widely. See Brown et al. (2002); Hunt, Arar, and Akana (2000); Johnson et al. (2006); Mikhail, Wali, and Ziment (2004); Pegado, Kwan, and Medeiros (2003); Poss, Jezewski, and Stuart (2003); Yeh et al. (2003); and Zaldivar and Smolowitz (1994).

8. City Terrace is an unincorporated community in eastern Los Angeles with a predominantly Latina/o population. Echo Park is in the central region of Los Angeles just west and slightly north of Downtown; 53 percent of residents are foreign born, of which most came from Mexico and El Salvador. Venice is on the west side of Los Angeles abutting the Pacific Ocean; about 22 percent of the population is foreign born, of which 38 percent is from Mexico. Culver City, containing a mixed population of which about one-fourth is of Mexican descent, lies east and south of Venice.

9. See also Geil and McWhorter (2008); Ghannam et al. (1986); Gutierrez (1998); Lopez (2007); Rodriguez-Fragoso et al. (2008); and Shapiro and Gong (2002).

10. The realization that behavior may be altered because individuals know they are being studied occurred during a research project (1927–1932) at the Hawthorne Plant of the Western Electric Company in Cicero, Illinois, which was led by Elton Mayo of the Harvard Business School.

11. For example, the kinds of interview guides suggested by James (2004) and Liburd (2003).

12. Indeed, having patients who are actively involved in their own care and treatment is a desirable outcome. If they are encouraged to be engaged, they make better patients overall (see Kitta 2012:137).

13. Olson, Sabogal, and Perez (2008); Ransford, Carrillo, and Rivera (2010).

14. This is a common complaint, suggesting that it is rarely addressed in intervention programs. See Adams (2003); von Goeler et al. (2003); Hatcher and Whittemore (2007); and Jezewski and Poss (2002). Quatromoni et al. (1994) write, "Overall, standard diet therapy for diabetes was regarded as unappealing, irrelevant, and unrelated to Latino culture and lifestyle" (871). As suggestions for future programs, the authors report that in focus groups, "There was widespread agreement that healthcare providers and nutritionists should learn more about the Latino culture, including folk remedies, dietary practices, and foods specific to their country of origin" (872).

References

Adams, Carmen Rivera. 2003. "Lessons Learned from Urban Latinas with Type 2 Diabetes Mellitus." *Journal of Transcultural Nursing* 14 (3):255–68.

Anderson, J. M., C. Blue, and A. Lau. 1991. "Women's Perspectives on Chronic Illness: Ethnicity, Ideology, and Restructuring of Life." *Social Science & Medicine* 32 (2):101–13.

Anderson, Robert M., and Martha M. Funnell. 2000. "Compliance and Adherence Are Dysfunctional Concepts in Diabetes Care." *Diabetes Educator* 26 (4):597–604.

Arcury, T. A., A. H. Skelly, W. M. Gesler, and M. C. Dougherty. 2004. "Diabetes Meanings among Those without Diabetes: Explanatory Models of Immigrant Latinos in Rural North Carolina." *Social Science & Medicine* 59 (11):2183–93.

Ashley, Bob, Joanne Hollows, Steve Jones, and Ben Taylor. 2004. *Food and Cultural Studies.* London: Routledge.

Beoku-Betts, Josephine A. 1995. "We Got Our Way of Cooking Things: Women, Food, and Preservation of Cultural Identity among the Gullah." *Gender and Society* 9 (5):535–55.

Bisogni, Carole A., Margaret Connors, Carol M. Devine, and Jeffery Sobal. 2002. "Who We Are and How We Eat: A Qualitative Study of Identities in Food Choice." *Journal of Nutrition Education and Behavior* 34 (3):128–40.

Brody, Gene H., Leonard Jack Jr., Velma McBride Murry, Melissa Lander-Potts, and Leandris Liburd. 2001. "Heuristic Model Linking Contextual Processes to Self-Management in African-American Adults with Type 2 Diabetes." *Diabetes Educator* 27 (5):685–93.

Broom, Dorothy, and Andrea Whittaker. 2004. "Controlling Diabetes, Controlling Diabetics: Moral Language in the Management of Diabetes Type 2." *Social Science & Medicine* 58 (11):2371–82.

Brown, Mary Helen de la Peña, 1981. "*Una Tamalada*: The Special Event." *Western Folklore* 40 (1):64–71.

Brown, Sharon A., Alexandra A. Garcia, Kamiar Kouzekanani, and Craig L. Hanis. 2002. "Culturally Competent Diabetes Self-Management Education for Mexican Americans: The Starr County Border Health Initiative." *Diabetes Care* 25 (2):259–68.

Caban, Arlene, and Elizabeth A. Walker. 2006. "A Systematic Review of Research on Culturally Relevant Issues for Hispanics with Diabetes." *Diabetes Educator* 32 (4):584–95.

Campbell, E. M., S. Redman, P. S. Moffitt, and R. W. Sanson-Fisher. 1996. "The Relative Effectiveness of Educational and Behavioral Instruction Programs for Patients with NIDDM: A Randomized Trial." *Diabetes Educator* 22 (4):379–86.

Coronado, G. D., B. Thompson. S. Tejeda, and R. Godina. 2004. "Attitudes and Beliefs among Mexican Americans about Type 2 Diabetes." *Journal of Health Care for the Poor and Underserved* 15 (4):576–88.

Counihan, Carole M. 1999. *The Anthropology of Food and Body: Gender, Meaning, and Power.* New York: Routledge.

Daniulaityte, Raminta. 2004. "Making Sense of Diabetes: Cultural Models, Gender and Individual Adjustment to Type 2 Diabetes in a Mexican Community." *Social Science & Medicine* 59 (9):1899–1912.

Davidhizar, R., G. Bechtel, and J. N. Giger. 1998. "When Your Client in the Surgical Suite Is Mexican American." *Today's Surgical Nurse* 20 (6):29–35.

Diamant, A. L., S. H. Babey, T. A. Hastert, and E. R. Brown. 2007. "Diabetes: The Growing Epidemic." *Policy Brief* (UCLA Center for Health Policy Research) (PB2007-9):1–12.

Douglas, Mary O. 1972. "Deciphering a Meal." *Daedalus* 101 (Winter):54–72.

Geil, Patti, and Laura Shane-McWhorter. 2008. "Dietary Supplements in the Management of Diabetes: Potential Risks and Benefits." *Journal of the American Dietetic Association* 108 (4):S59–S65.

Ghannam, N., M. Kingston, I. Al-Meshaal, M. Tarig, N. S. Parman, and N. Woodhouse. 1986. "The Antidiabetic Activity of Aloes: Preliminary Clinical and Experimental Observations." *Hormone Research* 24 (4):288–94.

Glasgow, R. E., and V. L. Osteen. 1992. "Evaluating Diabetes Education: Are We Measuring the Most Important Outcomes?" *Diabetes Care* 15 (10):1423–32.

Glazier, R. H., J. Bajcar, N. R. Kennie, and K. Wilson. 2006. "A Systematic Review of Interventions to Improve Diabetes Care in Socially Disadvantaged Populations." *Diabetes Care* 29 (7):1675–88.

Greene, Jessica, and Michael J. Yedidia. 2005. "Provider Behaviors Contributing to Self-Management of Chronic Illness among Underserved Populations." *Journal of Health Care for the Poor and Underserved* 16 (4):808–24.

Greenhalgh, T., C. Helman, and A. M. Chowdhury. 1998. "Health Beliefs and Folk Models of Diabetes in British Bangladeshis: A Qualitative Study." *British Medical Journal* 316 (7136):978–83.

Gutierrez, Miguel Angel. 1998. "Medicinal Use of the Latin Food Staple Nopales: The Prickly Pear Cactus." *Nutrition Bytes* 4 (2), Article 3, n.p. http://escholarship.org/uc/item/2x53d917.

Hall, Teri A. 1987. "Designing Culturally Relevant Education Materials for Mexican American Clients." *Diabetes Educator* 13 (3):281–85.

Hatcher, Erin, and Robin Whittemore. 2007. "Hispanic Adults' Beliefs about Type 2 Diabetes: Clinical Implications." *Journal of the American Academy of Nurse Practitioners* 19 (10):536–45.

Heisley, Deborah Dale. 1990. "Gender Symbolism in Food." PhD diss., Northwestern University.

Helton, L. R. 1996. "Folk Medicine and Health Beliefs: An Appalachian Perspective." *Journal of Cultural Diversity* 3 (4):123–28.

Hufford, David J. 1995. "Beings without Bodies: An Experience-Centered Theory of the Beliefs in Spirits." In *Out of the Ordinary: Folklore and the Supernatural*, ed. Barbara Walker, 11–45. Logan: Utah State University Press.

Hunt, Linda M., Miguel A. Valenzuela, and Jacquiline A. Pugh. 1997. "NIDDM Patients' Fears and Hopes about Insulin Therapy: The Basis of Patient Reluctance." *Diabetes Care* 20 (3):292–98.

———. 1998. "*Porque me tocó a mi?* Mexican American Diabetes Patients' Causal Stories and Their Relationship to Treatment Behaviors." *Social Science & Medicine* 46 (8):959–69.

Hunt, Linda M., N. H. Arar, and L. L. Akana. 2000. "Herbs, Prayer, and Insulin: Use of Medical and Alternative Treatments by a Group of Mexican American Diabetes Patients." *Journal of Family Practice* 49 (3):216–23.

Jack, Leonard, Jr. 2004. "Understanding the Environmental Issues in Diabetes Self-Management Education Research: A Reexamination of 8 Studies in Community-Based Settings." *Annals of Internal Medicine* 140 (11):964–72.

James, Delores C. S. 2004. "Factors Influencing Food Choices, Dietary Intake, and Nutrition-Related Attitudes among African Americans: Application of a Culturally Sensitive Model." *Ethnicity & Health* 9 (4):349–67.

Jezewski, Mary Ann, and Jane E. Poss. 2002. "Mexican Americans' Explanatory Model of Type 2 Diabetes." *Western Journal of Nursing Research* 24 (8):840–58.

Johnson, Lane, Hal Strich, Ann Taylor, Barbara Timmermann, Daniel Malone, Nicky Teufel-Shone, Rebecca Drummond, Raymond Woosley, Eladio Pereira, and Art Martinez. 2006. "Use of Herbal Remedies by Diabetic Hispanic Women in the Southwestern United States." *Phytotherapy Research* 20 (4):250–55.

Jonas, W. B., D. Eisenberg, D. Hufford, and C. Crawford. 2013. "The Evolution of Complementary and Alternative Medicine (CAM) in the USA over the Last 20 Years." *Forschende Komplementärmedizin* 20 (1):65–72.

Jones, Michael Owen. 2007. "Food Choice, Symbolism, and Identity: Bread-and-Butter Issues for Folklorists and Nutrition Studies." American Folklore Society Presidential Address, October 2005. *Journal of American Folklore* 120 (476):129–77.

Kerr, M., and N. Charles. 1986. "Servers and Providers: The Distribution of Food within the Family." *Sociological Review* 34 (1):115–57.

Kitta, Andrea. 2012. *Vaccinations and Public Concern in History: Legend, Rumor, and Risk Perception.* New York: Routledge.

Liburd, Leandris C. 2003. "Food, Identity, and African-American Women with Type 2 Diabetes: An Anthropological Perspective." *Diabetes Spectrum* 16 (3):160–66.

Loewe, Ron, and Joshua Freeman. 2000. "Interpreting Diabetes Mellitus: Differences between Patient and Provider Models of Disease and Their Implications for Clinical Practice." *Culture, Medicine and Psychiatry* 24 (4):379–401.

Lopez, Jose Luis, Jr. 2007. "Use of Opuntia Cactus as a Hypoglycemic Agent in Managing Type 2 Diabetes Mellitus among Mexican American Patients." *Nutrition Bytes* 12 (1):n.p.

Martínez, Iveris L., and Olivia Carter-Pokras. 2006. "Assessing Health Concerns and Barriers in a Heterogeneous Latino Community." *Journal of Health Care for the Poor and Underserved* 17 (4):899–909.

Mikhail, Nasser, Soma Wali, and Irwin Ziment. 2004. "Use of Alternative Medicine among Hispanics." *Journal of Alternative and Complementary Medicine* 10 (5):851–59.

Mull, Dorothy S., Nghia Nguyen, and J. Dennis Mull. 2001. "Vietnamese Diabetic Patients and Their Physicians: What Ethnography Can Teach Us." *Western Journal of Medicine* 175 (5):307–11.

Nabhan, Gary Paul. 1998. "Food, Health, and Native-American Farming and Gathering." In *Eating Culture*, ed. Ron Scapp and Brian Seitz, 169–79. Albany: State University of New York Press.

National Institutes of Health. 2005. "Diuretics Effective for People with Diabetes and High Blood Pressure." http://nih.gov/news/pr/jun2005/nhlbi-27.htm (accessed February 4, 2006).

Olson, Rebecca, Fabio Sabogal, and Ana Perez. 2008. "*Viva La Vida*: Helping Latino Medicare Beneficiaries with Diabetes Live Their Lives to the Fullest." *American Journal of Public Health* 98 (2):205–8.

Oomen, Jody S., Lynda J. Owen, and L. Suzanne Suggs. 1999. "Culture Counts: Why Current Treatment Models Fail Hispanic Women with Type 2 Diabetes." *Diabetes Educator* 25:220–25.

Pegado, Vance, Debbie Kwan, and Lina Medeiros. 2003. "'Do You Use Any Herbal Remedies?'—The Impact of Herbal Remedy Use on Diabetes Self-Management in Different Ethnic Groups." *University of Toronto Medical Journal* 80 (3):262–64.

Philis-Tsimikas, Athena, Chris Walker, Lena Rivard, Gregory Talavera, Joachim O. Reimann, Michelle Salmon, and Rachel Arujo. 2004. "Improvement in Diabetes Care of Underinsured Patients Enrolled in Project *Dulce*: A Community-based, Culturally Appropriate, Nurse Case Management and Peer Education Diabetes Care Model." *Diabetes Care* 27 (1):110–15.

Poss, Jane E., and Mary Ann Jezewski. 2002. "The Role and Meaning of Susto in Mexican Americans' Explanatory Model of Type 2 Diabetes." *Medical Anthropology Quarterly* 16 (3):360–77.

Poss, Jane E., Mary Ann Jezewski, and Armando Gonzalez Stuart. 2003. "Home Remedies for Type 2 Diabetes Used by Mexican Americans in El Paso, Texas." *Clinical Nursing Research* 12 (4):304–23.

Quatromoni, Paula A., Marian Milbauer, Barbara M. Posner, Nicolas Parkhurst Carballeira, Melanie Brunt, and Stuart R. Chipkin. 1994. "Use of Focus Groups to Explore Practices and Health Beliefs of Urban Caribbean Latinos with Diabetes." *Diabetes Care* 17 (8):869–73.

Ransford, H. Edward, Frank R. Carrillo, and Yessenia Rivera. 2010. "Health Care-Seeking Among Latino Immigrants: Blocked Access, Use of Traditional Medicine, and the Role of Religion." *Journal of Health Care for the Poor and Underserved* 21 (3):862–78.

Rock, Melanie. 2003. "Sweet Blood and Social Suffering: Rethinking Cause-Effect Relationships in Diabetes, Distress, and Duress." *Medical Anthropology* 22 (2):131–74.

Rodriguez-Fragoso, Lourdes, Jorge Reyes-Esparza, Scott Burchiel, Dea Herrera-Ruiz, and Eliseo Torres. 2008. "Risks and Benefits of Commonly Used Herbal Medicines in México." *Toxicology and Applied Pharmacology* 227 (1):125–35.

Rozin, Elisabeth. 1982. "The Structure of Cuisine." In *The Psychobiology of Human Food Selection*, ed. Lewis M. Barker, 189–203. Westport, CT: AVI.

Rubin, R. R., M. Peyrot, and C. D. Saudek. 1991. "Differential Effect of Diabetes Education on Self-regulation and Life-style Behaviors." *Diabetes Care.* 14 (4):335–38.

Schlundt, David G., Margaret K. Hargreaves, and Maciej S. Buchowski. 2003. "The Eating Behavior Patterns Questionnaire Predicts Dietary Fat Intake in African American Women." *Journal of the American Dietetic Association* 103 (3):338–45.

Schoenberg, N. E., E. M. Drew, E. P. Stoller, and C. S. Kart. 2005. "Situating Diabetes: Lessons from Lay Discourses on Diabetes." *Medical Anthropology Quarterly* 19 (2):171–93.

Shapiro, Karen, and William C. Gong. 2002. "Natural Products Used for Diabetes." *Journal of the American Pharmaceutical Association* 42 (2):217–26.

Sharman, Anne, Janet Theophano, Karen Curtis, and Ellen Messer. 1991. *Diet and Domestic Life in Society*. Philadelphia: Temple University Press.

Shelley, Brian M., Andrew L. Sussman, Robert L. Williams, Alissa R. Segal, and Benjamin F. Crabtree. 2009. "'They Don't Ask Me So I Don't Tell Them': Patient-Clinician Communication about Traditional, Complementary, and Alternative Medicine." *Annals of Family Medicine* 7 (2):139–47.

Sobal, Jeffrey. 2005. "Men, Meat, and Marriage: Models of Masculinity." *Food & Foodways* 13 (1–2):135–58.

Surwit, R. S., and M. S. Schneider. 1993. "Role of Stress in the Etiology and Treatment of Diabetes Mellitus." *Advances in Psychosomatic Medicine* 55 (4):380–93.

Surwit, R. S., and P. G. Williams. 1996. "Animal Models Provide Insight into Psychosomatic Factors in Diabetes." *Advances in Psychosomatic Medicine* 58 (6):582–89.

Tripp-Reimer, Toni, Eunice Choi, Lisa Skemp Kelley, and Janet C. Enslein. 2001. "Cultural Barriers to Care: Inverting the Problem." *Diabetes Spectrum* 14 (1):13–22.

Vandebroek, Ina, Victoria Reyes-García, Ulysses P de Albuquerque, Rainer Bussmann, and Andrea Pieroni. 2011. "Local Knowledge: Who Cares?" *Journal of Ethnobiology and Ethnomedicine* 7 (35): 1–7.

Vinicor, Frank, and Leonard Jack Jr. 2004. "25 Years and Counting: Centers for Disease Control and Prevention Identifies Opportunities and Challenges for Diabetes Prevention and Control." *Annals of Internal Medicine* 140 (11):943–44.

Visser, Margaret. 1986. *Much Depends on Dinner*. Toronto: McClelland and Stewart Weidenfeld.

von Goeler, Dorothea S., Milagros C. Rosal, Judith K. Ockene, Jeffrey Scavron, and Fernando De Torrijos. 2003. "Self-Management of Type 2 Diabetes: A Survey of Low-Income Urban Puerto Ricans." *Diabetes Educator* 29 (4):663–72.

Weller, S. C., R. D. Baer, L. M. Pachter, R. T. Trotter, M. Glazer, J. E. Garcia de Alba Garcia, and R. E. Klein. 1999. "Latino Beliefs about Diabetes." *Diabetes Care* 22 (5):722–28.

Whittemore, Robin. 2008. "Culturally Competent Interventions for Hispanic Adults with Type 2 Diabetes: A Systematic Review." *Journal of Transcultural Nursing* 18 (2):157–66.

Yeh, Gloria Y., David M. Eisenberg, Ted J. Kaptchuk, and Russell S. Phillips. 2003. "Systematic Review of Herbs and Dietary Supplies for Glycemic Control in Diabetes." *Diabetes Care* 26 (4):1277–94.

Zaldivar, A., and J. Smolowitz. 1994. "Perceptions of the Importance Placed on Religion and Folk Medicine by Non-Mexican-American Hispanic Adults with Diabetes." *Diabetes Educator* 20 (4):303–6.

CHAPTER FIVE

Interpreting and Treating Autism in Javanese Indonesia: Listening to Folk Perspectives on Developmental Difference and Inclusion

—Annie Tucker

Autism spectrum disorder (ASD) is a complex neurodevelopmental disability primarily affecting language, socialization, and behavior that is often accompanied by additional symptoms such as gastrointestinal dysfunction, sensorimotor differences, sleep disturbance, intellectual disability, seizures, and anxiety. As a spectrum disorder, autism affects people in different ways, with different combinations and severity of symptoms leading to a wide diversity of profiles. With an acknowledged genetic component but a still-contested etiology, autism has a fascinating history that has captured an exponentially growing clinical attention and vernacular imagination and spurred significant debate (Murray 2010). Even as much remains to be learned—or perhaps unlearned—about ASD, global interest in and diagnosis of autism continues to increase. Sociocultural research undertaken from Israel (Shaked and Bilu 2006) to India (Daley 2002) to South Africa (Grinker 2007) to South Korea (Grinker and Cho 2013) suggests that even as autism is an increasingly widespread, a globalized framework of interpretation for social and developmental differences, familiarity with ASD symptoms, and diagnosis varies widely. Meanwhile, local beliefs, practices, and concerns influence the way families interpret and respond to developmental difference and whether they see the diagnosis to be a good fit for their children.

Disabilities are constructed in a dialectical relationship with local ideas about personhood and well-being, parameters of normalcy, and available services (Ingstad and Whyte 1995; Skinner and Weisner 2007; Wendell 2000). Taking this into account, recent projects have scoured folklore and folk models of developmental difference for analogues to autism (Frith 2003; Leask, Leask, and Silove 2005), with implications for advocacy and policy. But while those with other central concerns have used folklore to search for autism, folklorists have been, with a few notable exceptions (Brady 2013; Eberly 1988; Kitta 2012; Shuman 2011, 2013) relatively quiet on the topic of autism and developmental disability, despite the fact that local "folk theories" (Daley and Weisner 2003) about healthy and delayed development may be implicated in various therapies or interventions (Daley 2004; Danesco 1997; Garcia, Perez, and Ortiz 2000; Kim 2012; Jegatheesan, Miller, and Fowler 2010; Levy et al. 2003; Ohta et al. 1987). Folkloristic perspectives have illuminated how communities respond to new diagnoses (Goldstein 2004), examined local interpretations for what could otherwise be called neuropsychiatric disorder (Etsuoko 1991), and used this understanding to inform effective syncretic treatment (Hufford 1998). A similar approach to studying ASD in different cultural places might prove similarly fruitful.

Autism Spectrum Disorder in Indonesia: A "New Phenomenon"

Java is Indonesia's most populous island, a historic and contemporary hub of government, education, and media production. Javanese people comprise over half the Indonesian population and are one of the largest ethnic groups in Southeast Asia (Sutarto 2007). Although there are an estimated one million autistic Indonesians, autism awareness in Java is considered a "new phenomenon" (Diniah 2010) paralleling a broader global history (Feinstein 2010) where the impetus for autism awareness and response initially came from parents who conducted independent research; traveled abroad to study psychology and special education; returned home to found activist, clinical, and service organizations, often inviting foreign specialists to consult; and compiled relevant libraries and materials. These grassroots efforts were important in spreading information about the label, criteria, and treatment of autism and inaugurating a public discussion about children with "special needs" (Tucker 2013). Slowly, state and private institutions have begun to assume greater responsibility for meeting these needs as sweeping economic, political, and social changes in the late twentieth and early twenty-first century led many parts of the country to new levels of stability, affluence, education, and good health (Vickers 2005).[1] Meanwhile, increasing Internet connectivity and growing numbers of transnational families have exposed Indonesians to the global disability rights movement and new information about child development.

Since the mid-1990s, autism has grown increasingly familiar across Indonesia as a clinical diagnosis and in popular culture. Outreach efforts continue at an increasingly robust pace, encompassing specialized lectures, panels, and workshops; public awareness events; newsletters and support groups; memoir; film; and journalistic coverage. Influenced by disparate fields from orthopedagogy to the self-advocacy movement, these efforts (re)introduce and (re)frame autism for participants, with the common crosscutting globalized model of ASD as a distinct neurodevelopmental disorder recognizable through certain signs and symptoms that requires proactive response and particular treatment to achieve best outcomes.

This model brings benefits to Javanese families. Despite its unfamiliarity, in some cases autism seems like a better fit than local explanatory models. Through autism awareness activities, parents can build networks of emotional and practical support, and with increased exposure and training, new programs can be established in communities where autistic children were previously without services. Concerned parties become empowered to further advocate for autistic people's rights. However, there are challenges as well. From the perspective of many activists and educators, there is an overwhelming lack of understanding about autism in Indonesia that they seek to remediate. Yet the new ideas they would disseminate—often couched in medicalized vocabulary, grounded in foreign paradigms of healthy development, and promoting unfamiliar psycho-educational and behavioral approaches—frequently conflict with local theories of healthy child development, practices of normative sociality, and responses to atypical behavior. In other words, there is in fact an understanding about autistic difference in Indonesia that must be accounted for by those who would aim to support and serve affected families.

Based on a year of exploratory multisited ethnographic fieldwork across Java, including interviews with family members of people diagnosed with autism, educators, activists, therapists, and clinicians[2]; observation, and participant observation of available treatments; and attendance at conferences, workshops, and awareness events, this chapter documents both folk and globalized biomedical and behavioral models of ASD in Javanese Indonesia; analyzes areas of friction between these; and introduces an experimental therapy that works with, rather than against, Javanese folk models of healthy development to quite promising effect.

Folk Labels and Treatments for Autistic Difference in Java

Javanese families reported a number of labels applied to their children by family or community members, both before and after diagnosis. The widely varied symptoms influenced the labels used. Being "in a world of one's own," crying or laughing with no apparent reason, wandering, and sensory hypersensitivity were labeled as crazy (*edan, gila*), a term typically reserved for severely disturbed people. Aggression or tantrums were often labeled as *ngamuk*, a laden cultural term reserved for violent outbursts. Alternately, such symptoms were taken to be signs of possession by a spirit (*kesambet, kesurupan*), not uncommon in Javanese ritual and everyday contexts. Poor impulse control and hyperactivity were called naughty (*nakal*). Challenges with self-care skills were labeled as delayed (*terlambat*) or stupid (*bodoh*), as was difficulty speaking, which was also sometimes confused with deaf-muteness (*tuli-bisu*).[3]

More often than not, parents perceived these local labels to be stigmatizing or inaccurate. For example, a father who knew his son to be alert, considerate, and with a photographic memory of the family record collection despite his social limitations and occasional severe outbursts, could not accept that he was, as friends and family called him, crazy or stupid. A mother who knew her nonverbal son struggled to communicate his intentions was deeply hurt when another family called him naughty for scratching their daughter on the playground. A third parent, who knew her daughter fretted if the television was turned off, even if she was in another room, couldn't believe that she was deaf. However, parents, knowing of no other local label that was a better fit, were left wondering. Thus, in the midst of multiple folk understandings of developmental differences, ASD could be a welcome alternative.

Javanese families sought a range of folk and alternative treatments to ameliorate symptoms, including home remedies eaten to stimulate speech; herbal tonics (*jamu*) and massage (*pijat*), which both play a significant role in Javanese traditional health care and preventative medicine; acupuncture, acupressure, and reflexology, also widespread; and the rarer *balur*, which combines massage, smoke baths, and topical exfoliants and suppositories made from various ingredients such as vitamin C or garlic paste to detoxify the body. An underlying logic unifying these therapies is the Javanese conception of health wherein the body is made up of channels (*aliran*) of energy, humors, or bodily fluids that should flow freely. Illness may be caused by a buildup of toxins that block such flows, with health restored by breaking these toxins down (Ferzacca 2001). This indigenous philosophy of health logically aligns with one (contested but still prevalent) theory of autism that posits its etiology in the buildup of heavy metals, chemicals, or other toxins inside the body.

Beyond tending to the body, many families also sought the assistance of traditional healers (*dukun*) who diagnose and advise on supernatural matters. For example, a *dukun* told one mother a malevolent spirit possessed her daughter and recommended a ritual wherein the spirit could be transferred into a goat, which could then be slaughtered, freeing the girl. Another *dukun* diagnosed an autistic boy as a victim of black magic sent by his father's jealous colleague. Islamic families may seek faith-based intervention, such as Koran recitation or consultation with a spiritual adviser (*kyai*).

Clearly, there are a variety of options open to families seeking treatment for children exhibiting autistic symptoms. These will be the only treatments some Javanese ever receive, in part because specialized interventions are geographically and financially inaccessible to many. Those families who *do* have access to other therapies may still continue to pursue folk and alternative treatments because they address spiritual factors that medical and psychoeducational treatments cannot and also provide sensory-rich and intersubjective work toward cure (Jones et al. 2001; O'Connor and Hufford 2001).

"I Thought of My Child as Normal": The Complexities of Autism Recognition and Response in a Local Cultural Context

Just as scholars have sought autism in folklore, hoping to make it transculturally and historically visible, Indonesian autism awareness advocates (Sarasvati 2004) often try to teach parents how to "see" autism by providing a checklist of the classical signs used in clinical screening instruments (a lack of eye contact, absence of pointing, apparent nonresponsiveness to social cues, etc.). The assumption is that if Javanese parents know these signs, they will recognize autism and thus respond with intervention and treatment in a fairly straightforward manner. However, narratives shared by parents suggested that the lived realities of autism recognition might be more complicated.

Interpreting a Quiet Baby: A Sign of Precocious Maturity or Autistic Pathology?

Sri Murni lives in Semarang, a large city on the northern coast of Central Java. With modest finances, Murni used to work at a drink stand while raising her two children. She remembers her reactions to her infant son Faisal's behavior:

> I would lay my little one down in a crib . . . and start to boil water to make *es lilin* [the drink I sold in the market]. When I did that, Faisal really helped me out because he rarely cried. "Father, our child is so smart, you know! He's never cranky, even when I leave him alone," I said.
>
> But when he was 2.8 years old, he began to show signs of unusual development, different from his older sister. Because Faisal never cried except when he had peed or to ask for milk, I thought he was so smart, so sweet, and so well behaved . . . well it turns out, I was wrong!

Parents anticipate the expression of culturally valued ways of behaving and project these values onto the behaviors of their infants, which is itself an enculturating process (Keller 2007). In her story, Sri remembers interpreting Faisal's low interactivity as precociously considerate and calm, viewing his behavior through the lens of Javanese cultural values that emphasize an ideology of interdependence where harmony (*rukun*), intuition (*rasa*), and the ability to suppress one's own desires for the good of the collective (*ngalah*) are emphasized, and therefore self-effacement and an unwillingness to directly assert one's needs are prized qualities of comportment (Geertz 1961; Keeler 1983; 1987; Subandi 2009). Indeed, Sri felt her son was exhibiting a remarkable maturity in understanding that her need to work uninterrupted for the good of the family was more important than his need for the kind of attention typical infants require; hence she approved of his behavior.

However, at the time of this telling, Faisal was already an adolescent; after years of struggle with her son and deep involvement in the autism world, Sri Murni has learned that low interactivity in infancy may be one of the earliest manifestations of the autistic impairment of socialization and communication skills that her son later exhibited (Glickman 2013; Kanner 1943). Sri Murni has thus experienced a significant paradigm shift and now sees her initial, Javanese interpretation as misguided: rather than being "smart, sweet, and well-behaved," her son was exhibiting signs of developmental disability.[4]

Avoiding Labels and Postponing Specialized Interventions: Irresponsible Neglect or Adaptive Inclusion?

Even when Javanese parents notice their child exhibiting troubling—not precocious—atypical behavior, they may still choose to interpret this as personal idiosyncrasy and think of the child as "normal." Warno is from Salatiga, an inland town in Central Java. After his wife died, Warno noted certain changes in the youngest of his three sons. Three-year-old Asto wasn't speaking, didn't react when his name was called, refused to eat anything except instant noodles, and was distressed by loud noises. Warno interpreted this as the reaction of a grieving son who needed extra care and attention, which he strove to provide. As Asto grew and his symptoms did not subside, Warno saved up to take him to Jakarta for evaluation. Asto was diagnosed with autism, but Warno could not afford ongoing treatment in Jakarta, and there were few autism services in his area. So he rejected the diagnosis, saying, "I had a principle. Because his older brothers were normal, I looked at my child as normal and I treated him as if he was normal." Warno homeschooled Asto for almost a decade until a school for children with autism opened near his house and offered him a scholarship. While Asto soon caught up with his peers academically, his new teachers scolded Warno for not seeking out education or therapy earlier, bemoaning the lost opportunities that might have taken the bright Asto even further while suggesting that such a normalizing or slow response is at best ignorant and at worse willfully neglectful. However, Warno's may not be an unusual response for Javanese parents with young children ultimately diagnosed with autism—and the way Warno sees it, his patience bore fruit.

Patience (*sabar*) is a core virtue and a common response to neuropsychiatric disorder in Javanese culture (Lemelson 2011; Sutarto 2007). According to a philosophy of *sabar*, the vagaries of fate are mysterious and out of individual control, due to karmic retribution or divine trial. As such, the best thing to do is to manage negative feelings or desire for specific outcomes and have faith that meaning, positive change, or divine reward will come in time (Geertz 1970; Goddard 2001). Patience is hence temporal, psychological, and spiritual, and as much directed inward toward the parent as outward toward the child with autism. Patience thus understood is a distinctly Javanese coping strategy when compared to, for example, the responses of contemporary Californian-American mothers to a similar diagnosis. As described in Lappe (2013), these mothers reacted with a sense of anticipatory vigilance, preferring urgent early intervention and a preemptive modulation of the environment rather than a patient receptivity toward the future. This understanding of time as "running out" is one espoused by many autism awareness educators yet may be a particularly Western approach (Helman 1987).

There may be some benefits to "not seeing" autistic difference, particularly because in particular cultural contexts, nonclinical labels for difference allow parents to preserve a sense of full value of their children and normalcy for their family (Grinker and Cho 2013; Kapp 2011). Echoing Warno, a soft-spoken mother of a three-year-old from the city of Solo, who was also diagnosed in Jakarta, described her and her husband's approach: "We keep the situation from all our family. We care about [our son] and if everybody thinks he's a strange one . . . we don't want that. We still want him to be normal, and we keep telling him that he's a normal kid." She continued: "We as parents can't push him to do what we want. We just give him the chance, and whatever we have to help him grow into himself. And we keep telling him that he is special, that's what he needs. And giving him love, and keep him safe, as long as he needs. That is the most important."

Based on these recounted experiences, Javanese parents may not be seeing the early signs of autism as such; due to Javanese ideals of comportment and sociality, low interactivity may be viewed positively as good behavior, not as a preverbal clinical sign of any developmental problems. Even when certain symptoms are found to be troublesome, a diagnosis may still be eschewed and specialized treatment postponed. Instead, as parents assess behavior based on local understandings of development and determine what will best support their child's and their family's inclusion in a Javanese cultural context that values group harmony and avoids openly acknowledging family problems (Mulder 1994; Subandi 2011), they may patiently wait for change, particularly if there is little infrastructure or cultural context for autism treatment and the label is of minimal practical use. The principle of normalizing autistic behavior, minimizing differences, and explaining those differences as quirks within the context of the vagaries of family life while sheltering the child from potentially hurtful exchanges with outsiders and patiently adjusting expectations and adapting child-rearing strategies might therefore be considered a local model of adaptive inclusion that allows a family to avoid embarrassment, social stigma, and the financial burden of specialized care.

These culturally syntonic interpretations and locally adaptive approaches may come at a cost, in that they militate against early detection and intervention, which specialists assert are crucial for optimal long-term prognosis (Matson and Konst 2013). However, in taking these costs seriously and trying to emphasize a different orientation toward symptoms of difference, interventionists risk alienating or further worrying the families they are trying to help.

The "Wrong Kind of Love": Questioning Javanese Family Practices in the Context of Globalized Autism Intervention

Much of the information interventionists have about the signs and symptoms of autism as well as best practices in treatment were gained abroad in Australia, the United States, or the Netherlands or from specialists trained in these countries. This lends a particular perspective on socialization and behavior that might be different from, or perhaps even at odds with, the various local child-rearing methods with which parents feel more comfortable. The different interpretive lens of globalized autism intervention versus Javanese theories of development determine the preferred practices intended to promote the health and adaptive development of the autistic person, leading to charged debates about the "right" way to parent an autistic child.

For example, Gayatri Pramoedji, founder of the Autism Society of Indonesia, was a hotelier before her son was diagnosed with autism, which changed the course of her life. She went to study with behaviorists and special education experts in Australia, where her son was receiving therapy, and earned a master's degree in health counseling. Committed to disseminating interventions she learned abroad, she told me with some exasperation, "I haven't been able to find out the key to behavior change. And I'm not referring to the children here, that part's actually easy! I'm talking about the key to behavior change for Indonesian parents!" Here Gayatri refers to the parental behaviors required to implement the interventions she is recommending, including behavior therapy and biomedical treatment.[5] In prosperous urban areas of Java, where specialized autism interventions are available, these are among those commonly recommended, often in concert, and often meeting the most ambivalence and resistance.

Behavioral Approaches to Kids with Autism: Providing Necessary Structure or Exacerbating Harm?

Behavioral approaches, particularly those espoused in applied behavioral analysis (ABA), are some of the most frequently used treatments for autism in the United States and elsewhere (Myers and Johnson 2007). There is an extensive literature on the complex field of behavioral therapy science, but briefly, ABA aims to reduce problematic behaviors—such as aggression or repetitive movements—and teach socially adaptive ones, including school and self-care skills, through the antecedents and responses to those behaviors via punishments (e.g., saying "no," giving a "time out") or rewards (e.g., verbal praise, access to desired activity).[6] Developed through clinical testing in the United States, ABA treatment began as a preferred alternative to institutionalization for severely disabled children (Lovaas 1987). It has since been adapted to everyday settings, but consistency in enforcement remains a core principle; in order to predict and reshape behavior, reliable schedules and scripts of responses to behavior across a range of interactions must be provided (Knapp and Turnbull 2014). In ABA, compliance is required before other skills can be taught, and children are incrementally challenged to develop their capacities. Therefore, authority figures set rules and expectations with the understanding that when motivated by reward and deterred by punishment, children will practice and master ever more difficult skills, aligning with so-called common sense models of Euro-American parenting and learning, including an understanding that "power struggles" (Hoffman 2013) and a "generative tension" (Rothbaum et al. 2000) are both typical and potentially instructive aspects of parent-child relationships and maturational processes.

Susana, part of a Javanese family living on the island of Kalimantan, brought her five-year-old nephew Andi to Jakarta to receive ABA therapy at a specialized clinic in early 2012. Susana had been trying to implement ABA at home, but not everyone in the extended family household adhered to the program. She described how "because of too much love and too much pity we spoon feed him, we dress him, serve him, and fulfill all his needs, and that does not make him independent." Echoing Gayatri, she felt all the family members needed "some kind of therapeutic intervention to change their behavior."

The "Javanese cultural psychology" (Good, Subandi, and Good 2007) emphasizes the importance of balanced and pleasant states in maintaining a healthy mind and body. Negative states such as fear, shock, disappointment, anger, strain, and frustration weaken the essential life force, causing significant vulnerability to sickness, mental illness, spirit possession, and even death (Browne 2001; Ferzacca 2001; Subandi 2009). Infants and children are considered especially vulnerable, and many customs of child care are intended to protect against these and other unpleasant sensations (Geertz 1961; 1968), which can endanger the child's well-being "quite radically" (Keeler 1983:154). As such, many Javanese caregivers are uncomfortable denying children their desires, and in the case of conflict or difficulty prefer to defer to the child and support children in learning at their own pace (Geertz 1967). This "indulgent" attitude toward a young child is also instructional, stimulating a sense of indebtedness toward elder beneficiaries and teaching older siblings how to assume the benefactor role within such interdependent hierarchical relationships thought to strengthen family ties and facilitate group harmony within the wider Javanese social world (Ambarini 2006; Keeler 1983, 1987).

In circumstances where a child or even an older adult is exhibiting signs of significant disturbance or distress, this protective approach may be amplified or extended indefinitely through the process of "caring for gently" (*ngemong*) (Subandi 2011). Ngemong entails tolerating improper behavior, abstaining from criticism, and fulfilling needs with no expectations in return. When compared to *ngemong*, some Javanese parents see the ABA approach as at best unkind, at worst like "torture."[7] But once exposed to behavioral therapies, and the criticism of interventionists, some families are left wondering whether they are expressing the right kind of care or are damaging the autistic child's later chances at healthy functioning. They worry, as Susana worried: "How long can we act like this? What happens if he gets to be twelve years old and he can't do anything for himself? We are afraid." Providing the discipline and encouraging the independence autistic children seem to need goes against familiar norms of childrearing, and such a counterintuitive effort only becomes more complicated in situations of extended family living, shared child care, and the inevitable disruptions and changes in family life.

Restricted Diets as Treatment for ASD: Restoring Health or Withholding Affection?

Pando is a nine-year-old boy whose family has moved back home to Yogyakarta after challenging early years of frequent relocations due to his father's military assignments. The family has now settled into a routine that they believe is supporting Pando's development. They also attribute recent strides to his restricted diet. They didn't always follow this diet—his mother explains, "Since we didn't know our child was autistic, we *forced* him to snack, you know, fried chicken, fried noodles . . . even though he didn't want to. But we thought at that time—classic!—that little kids have to snack. It turns out we were wrong!" An older brother of one of Pando's classmates at a private school for students with autism added that he and his family also tend to overfeed his brother, now a strapping teenager, saying they do it because "It's the feeling of indulging. Feeling that he is protected by my mom and dad, feeling like he is being noticed and taken care of."

Foodways are often highly symbolic and contribute to child socialization by communicating cultural values, indicating and instructing in aspects of social relationships, and transmitting sentiment.[8] Foodways are also often tied to significant aspects of health and development in the context of autism. Biomedical treatment for ASD recommends a stringently restricted diet—avoiding gluten, casein, sugar, chemical additives, and a host of other foods depending on the child's profile—and a regimen of vitamins and supplements, with the belief that symptoms are caused or exacerbated by food allergies, difficulty digesting and processing certain proteins, or a physiological response to other substances in the body (White 2003). This approach remains scientifically unproven but has strong anecdotal support and is promoted and pursued in and outside of Java.

From a biomedical perspective, a restricted diet supports the autistic child by eliminating toxins from the body and ameliorating the ensuing discomfort and/or physical dysregulation. It also restores control to parents, who would otherwise be left guessing what was wrong with their child and trying to mitigate the symptoms—such as anxiety, irritation, or hyperactivity—that result from eating improper foods. Meanwhile, Javanese parents often believe that frequent snacking supports children's health. They are reassured by plumpness, which in a holistic conception of the body-mind indicates happiness and relaxation (Ferzacca 2001). Frequent snacking prevents states of discomfort or frustration and promotes interdependence, at once anticipating the needs of the child being fed and enforcing the will of the parents doing the feeding. Finally, snacks communicate attention and affection. This sentiment is so strong that some awareness advocates use strong language to combat it. For example, one workshop leader coined the phrase "autism *halal*" and "autism *haram*" for her predominantly Muslim attendees, equating the restricted autism diet to the holy diet allowed by the Koran and other foods to supposedly sinful foods like pork, which one must never even touch, telling me that when it comes to Javanese foodways, "These parents say, 'Love is food and food is love.' But love is an excuse."

Some parents, like Pando's mother, overcome their initial food logic to adopt restricted diets they believe are beneficial. From other Javanese parents' perspective, however, these diets seemed to make children grow sorrowfully skinny and feel excluded. They also made life challenging for the family, preventing the consumption of some of the most commonly consumed ingredients in Indonesian cuisine, such as soy sauce and sugar, forbidding Javanese favorites (such as fried chicken and fried noodles), and recommending the use of specialty food products that are hard to find and sometimes ten times more expensive than typical products. Yet with the sometime-proselytizing approach of restricted diet proponents, such mothers are left feeling like they have sinned against their children.

In sum, food is part of a local cultural and familial identity redolent with sentiment and social meaning, from which the child on a special diet is in part cut off. Food may play an even more significant role than usual for families who may have difficulty communicating with their autistic child verbally. For them, it is an act of love to feed their child delicious foods to communicate their nurturing and support; but again, via a biomedical perspective on autism intervention, Javanese caregivers are being convinced that theirs is the wrong kind of love.

What does a child need to grow up healthy: indulgence, protection, and support or challenges, rules, and restrictions? How should parents react to developmental difficulty: with patience or proactive intervention? Is snacking on Javanese foods healthy or harmful? Should you be proud of or worried about a quiet baby? Clearly, the answers to these questions depend on who is being asked, which leads to next set of questions: Should biomedical and behavioral theories, tested (and contested) in the West, automatically be used in Javanese families? What should be done if folk theories of disability position certain globalized autism interventions as potentially harmful to Javanese children, and vice versa?

The responses to autism by many professionals and advocates in the field seem to involve attempts to acculturate families out of local values and practices, attempts that are understandably challenging and often unsustainable (Weisner 1996). By not recognizing folk models of development, developmental difference, and inclusion as such—by dismissing them as simply misguided or as excuses—interventionists and advocates miss chances to develop successful interventions that might work with many Javanese families. This suggests a need for accessible and culturally coherent interventions for autistic Indonesians and their families and raises the possibility that locally guided and grounded practices of encouraging growth and development might point toward powerful therapeutic alternatives.

"If You Use Art, It Just Happens Spontaneously": Therapeutic Gamelan as Complementary Autism Intervention

The therapeutic gamelan group of Bina Anggita Autism School in Yogyakarta, Central Java, is an exciting and investigative effort innovated at the intersection of the comparatively new globalized diagnosis of autism and a long-standing Javanese musical heritage.

A gamelan is a percussion ensemble composed primarily of variously sized metallophones, gongs, and drums. Present in regional variation throughout Indonesia, gamelan is a potent symbol of Javanese identity depicted on the walls of the world-famous Borobudur temple, a ubiquitous accompaniment to significant civic and cultural events on the island for over twelve centuries thought to illustrate "the life journey of humankind" through personal development and public life (see Kodrat 1982; Susteya 2007). Gamelan ensembles are handled respectfully, cherished over multiple generations, lavished with titles such as "The Foremost and Venerable Harmonious Dragon" (Prijosusilo 2011) and sometimes believed to have supernatural powers. As a gamelan teacher told me, "In the olden days the king would say 'If my child can't play gamelan, I will not recognize him as my own.' Gamelan *is* Java."

Gamelan instruments are available in most villages and are a part of the public school curricula. They are believed to provide a profoundly integrating cultural-social-spiritual education based on a Javanese philosophy of personal and interpersonal development encouraging values of magnanimity, creativity, intelligence, and cooperation (Khisbiyah 2004:149). According to some, its structure is founded on the broadest possible inclusion and accord, so that "any group, including people of any age, gender or ability, can be guided in worshipfulness and harmony" (Prijosusilo 2011). And yet the idea for a gamelan orchestra comprised of autistic musicians is new. Budi Raharja, an ethnomusicology professor and gamelan instructor, developed the idea and created a modified gamelan by reducing the number of instruments to those easiest to play, scaling the instruments down in size, and painting them with kid-friendly designs. Twice a week for an hour and a half, students practice popular songs, taking turns introducing compositions and singing lead vocals with teachers assisting as needed. Teachers and parents reported that the multiple benefits of these sessions include a relaxed mood; improved social skills through practicing appropriate manners and speech when singing and introducing songs; improved ability to synchronize with others; improved cognitive skills through the memorization of and concentration on music; and improved motor skills, honed through physically playing the instruments.[9]

Regular performance is an important part of the gamelan program that is thought to bring its own benefits by breaking down stereotypes about autistic individuals and shifting the focus from the children's deficits to their abilities and potential. Since they began in 2009, the group has performed at numerous prestigious universities in Indonesia and for national television (TVRI). On a more intimate scale, seeing their children perform provides parental consolation and engagement. As one mother described the experience: "It's like when the doctor says that you cannot get pregnant, and then suddenly you're pregnant! The feeling is extraordinary."

Therapeutic gamelan may be successful as an intervention in part because it evokes Javanese values and beliefs about art, growth, and well-being. The performing arts have historically played an integral role in Javanese society, supported by a complex indigenous philosophy of intertwining ethics and aesthetics, recognized as bridging the sacred and the secular to express a uniquely Javanese way of being-in-the-world that might have key protective, curative, and restorative properties (Foley 1984; Woodward 1985). Faith healing, ritual, and folk treatments may be successful dynamic agents of change at the intersection of the sacred and the secular because they derive from, draw upon, and perform or embody cultural values, symbols, and beliefs (Santino 1985; Toelken 2001). Recent research into the growing field of medical ethnomusicology has elaborated on how similar dynamics might be enacted through musical practice and performance (Koen 2008). Gamelan performance in particular may serve as an embodied pneumonic for the social and spiritual values of inclusive diversity, harmonious cooperation, and tolerant community that Javanese Indonesians try to cultivate, and extend these in a new context of autistic difference.[10] As one audience member saw it, the message of the Bina Anggita gamelan is, "Come on, let's support one another, give to one another, accept one another. Diversity is an inherent part of humanity." Through therapeutic gamelan practice and performance, Javanese personhood is triggered within the audience members and read onto gamelan players, as can be illustrated through the story of one young student, Arka.

Arka's Growth: Achieving a Javanese Maturity through Javanese Means

Arka is a slim and soft-spoken teenager. Anis, a senior teacher at the school who plays a key role in organizing gamelan activities, noted significant changes in Arka's personality since he began playing with the school group: "Before he joined he . . . didn't want to socialize with other people, his emotions were out of control. Praise God, after he joined there have been a number of observable changes, like he wants to talk to other people even if he is slow to read their signals, his emotions have become controlled; he's starting to joke around with his friends." Yasin, the school's founder, added that "Arka has become more mature, more regulated, and his emotions are peaceful. He cares about others and he can lead the younger children. He offers to help the teachers . . . many positive behaviors have appeared since he has been participating in gamelan therapy." Arka's teachers describe the Javanese qualities of mature personhood they believe have been cultivated and drawn out by gamelan practice. Furthermore, they say Arka enjoyed the practice at school so much that for the first time he spoke up spontaneously and asked his parents to buy him one of the instruments, a *saron*, to practice with at home—a testament to gamelan's power to encourage engagement and self-expression.

Budi describes at length gamelan's unique ability to foster individual confidence and character through positive mind states leading to such a spontaneous individual initiative within the safe buffer of a supportive collective. He says,

> In gamelan, creativity is wide open. With the understanding that with creativity, within the scope of the rules, there is independence. The interaction between members is very flexible. So it's that, it's actually that *freedom* that I want to use to bolster and awaken the children's feelings so that they can create. . . . If you use art, they don't feel like they are being "treated." It just happens spontaneously because they are engaged.
>
> My assumption is that, if people play music they have to be happy first. If they are already happy [positive changes] will emerge on their own. It doesn't have to be like this [mimics a strict teacher scolding]. With that understanding, I made a gamelan that could be appropriate to their world.

Ultimately, the Javanese are working with different folk theories of healthy development than Euro-Americans, and these different theories are reflected and instantiated in models of autism intervention, which envision the healthy developing body differently. ABA theorizes the autistic child as learning to obey rules and scripts with the hopes of personal reward, trained to respond to ever-increasing demands. The biomedical diet theorizes the autistic body as becoming ever more restricted in order to stay healthy. These models are not so different from normative ideas about functional personhood and physical health in the contemporary United States but may feel counterintuitive or punitive to Javanese families. Meanwhile, the therapeutic gamelan imagines the healthy autistic body as a porous member of a collective who aligns in harmony with others, the healthy autistic child as flexible and agreeable, spontaneously expressing himself/herself when happy. This, too, is not far away from the Javanese ideal.

While it does not supplant the need for other treatments or services, therapeutic gamelan should be of interest to those looking to explore options for culturally coherent autism intervention in Javanese Indonesia. As yet unique, such groups could be replicated and such techniques applied more widely, at the very least throughout Java and Bali. Furthermore, just as Western-innovated interventions are being globally disseminated, so could effective local interventions. Research in medical ethnomusicology suggests that the accessibility of the instruments and the synchronized interaction that gamelan music facilitates provides benefits for players with disabilities when practiced outside the culture that shaped it (Bakan et al. 2008; MacDonald, O'Donnell, and Davies 1999; McIntosh 2005; Sanger and Kippen 1987), some of which can be traced through psychometric testing.[11]

Conclusion

Autistic difference is a newly available globalized interpretive framework for behavioral and development difference for Javanese families encompassing etiology, symptom, and response that might clash with or complement long-held beliefs and preferred practices regarding healthy and unusual development, some of which have been discussed here. Because autism is so complex—leading to various physical, emotional, developmental, and cognitive differences—parents call upon folk theories of development, health, personhood, and sociality that touch upon multiple arenas of daily life, including foodways, child rearing, sociality, religious faith, and the arts. The practices and institutions that have enabled the diagnosis and specialized treatment of autism in Indonesia are historically specific, variably salient and available, and yet ultimately gaining force. The ability to incorporate and address these multiple folk perspectives on developmental difference and inclusion will be crucial to providing effective, locally coherent, and galvanizing autism response in Indonesia and to developing practical and successful intervention, education, and treatment policy.

Finally, challenges in Java prove instructive when looking at ASD in other cultural places. Ultimately, in Java, when folk beliefs, values, and practices clash with the philosophies underlying proposed interventions for people with autism, the result can be confusion, conflict, or distress. However, if and when they are brought into harmony, new possibilities for the inclusion of people with ASD, family satisfaction, and locally innovated efficacious therapies emerge. The same theoretical model used to identify gamelan as therapy could also be employed to target or develop local interventions in other cultures and contexts. Would-be interventionists should look for activities that are readily familiar, available, and adaptable and therefore disseminated easily. They should look for community-supported activities that espouse local values and trigger feelings of positive inclusion and cultural pride, most probably those that incorporate elements of folk belief, folk practice, or folk healing. In other words, they should strive to capitalize on local strengths rather than try to change local culture (Brady 2001; Goldstein 2004; Hufford 1997; Kitta 2012; O'Connor 1995). Such parameters might be used to identify accessible, culturally logical interventions that are both symbolically and empirically efficacious in promoting personal development and social inclusion for people with autism. Furthermore, such parameters encourage the recognition of indigenous practices of inclusion, affection, patience, acceptance, hope, and growth in the context of developmental difference rather than a mere absence of autism awareness.

Notes

1. See Nadesan (2005) on similar developments in the United States and effects on autism recognition and response.

2. Core group N=30 family members of children aged 3 to 19 professionally diagnosed with autism. Interviews incorporated one or more family members and lasted one to four hours, were audio recorded as permitted and transcribed verbatim with field notes taken during and following all interviews. Research protocol and instruments were approved by UCLA's Institutional Review Board, study number 10-000680. All instruments were translated into Indonesian and verified by a professional interpreter. In order to protect respondents' privacy, first-name pseudonyms are used for those parents who have not already chosen to publicly share their stories as awareness advocates. This research was in part made possible by a Lemelson Fellowship for Indonesian Studies and a grant from the United States–Indonesia Society (USINDO).

3. Repetitive behaviors and restricted routines were noted but given no local label in isolation.

4. Sri Murni's interpretation of her quiet son was further influenced by a belief that boys speak later than girls. Other folk theories of delayed speech attest that children who walk or whose teeth grow in comparatively early will talk later than their peers (see Tucker 2013).

5. Note that the term *biomedical treatment* takes on a specific meaning in the autism context, which is different than the meaning generally used in CAM and Folk Medicine, as described in the following section of this essay.

6. In early ABA, electric shock was used as punishment (see "Screams, Slaps, and Love" article in *Life* Magazine, http://neurodiversity.com/library_screams_1965.html). Corporal aversives are no longer standard practice but are occasionally used in Indonesia, such as forcing the child to eat a chili pepper.

7. Even in North America, some have protested ABA for being punitive of autistic people, as in Michelle Dawson's influential 2004 online piece, "The Misbehavior of Behaviorists," http://www.sentex.net/~nexus23/naa_aba.html.

8. For an excellent review of the rich symbolism of foodways, see Jones (2007).

9. For a comprehensive list of benefits, see Tucker (2013).

10. Other performing arts have also been reported as beneficial. For example, see the article in the esteemed national newspaper *Kompas*, "Kuncir Recovers from Autism after Discovering *Wayang* [Shadow Puppetry]." Online version available at http://entertainment .kompas.com/read/2008/07/14/21410019/kuncir.sembuh.dari.autis.setelah.kenal.wayang.

11. See description of ongoing research at The Gamelan Project's webpage at The Temporal Dynamics of Learning Center at UCSD. http://tdlc.ucsd.edu/gamelan (accessed July 13, 2014).

References

Afflictions: Culture and Mental Illness in Indonesia. Directed by Robert Lemelson. 2010. Boston: Documentary Educational Resources, 2013. Film.

Ambarini, Tri Kurniati. 2006. "Saudara Sekandung Dari Anak Autis dan Peran Mereka Dalam Terapi." *Insan* 8 (2):112–35.

Bakan, Michel B., Benjamin Koen, Fred Kobylarz, Lindee Morgan, Rachel Goff, Sally Kahn, and Megan Bakan. 2008. "Following Frank: Respons-Ability and the Co-Creation of Culture in a Medical Ethnomusicology Program for Children on the Autism Spectrum." *Ethnomusicology* 52 (2):163–202.

Brady, Erika. 2001. *Healing Logics: Culture and Medicine in Modern Health Belief Systems*. Logan: Utah State University Press.

———. 2013. "Teaching Ethnographic Skills to University Students on the Autism Spectrum." Paper presented at the Annual Meeting of the American Folklore Society, Providence, RI, October 16–19.

Browne, Kevin O. 2001. "*(Ng)amuk* Revisited: Emotional Expression and Mental Illness in Central Java, Indonesia." *Transcultural Psychiatry* 38 (2):147–65.

Daley, Tamara Cohen. 2002. "The Need for Cross-Cultural Research on the Pervasive Developmental Disorders." *Transcultural Psychiatry* 39 (4):531–50.

———. 2004. "From Symptom Recognition to Diagnosis: Children with Autism in Urban India." *Social Science & Medicine* 58 (7):1323–35.

Daley, Tamara, and Thomas Weisner. 2003. "'I Speak a Different Dialect': Teen Explanatory Models of Difference and Disability." *Medical Anthropology Quarterly* 17 (1):25–48.

Danesco, Evangeline R. 1997. "Parental Beliefs on Childhood Disability: Insights on Culture, Child Development and Intervention." *International Journal of Disability, Development, and Education* 44 (1):41–52.

Diniah, Kholifatut. 2010. "Strategi Penanganan Anak Autis." Presentation at the Regional Seminar and Workshop on Getting a Handle on Autism, Salatiga, Central Java, Indonesia, August 1.

Eberly, Susan Schoon. 1988. "Fairies and the Folklore of Disability: Changelings, Hybrids, and the Solitary Fairy." *Folklore* 99 (1):58–77.

Feinstein, Adam. 2010. *A History of Autism: Conversations with the Pioneers*. Sussex, UK: Wiley Blackwell.

Ferzacca, Steve. 2001. *Healing the Modern in a Central Javanese City*. Durham, NC: Carolina Academic Press.

Foley, Kate. 1984. "Of *Dalang* and *Dukun*—Spirits and Men: Curing and Performance in the *Wayang* of West Java." *Asian Theater Journal* 1 (1):52–69.

Frith, Uta. 2003. *Autism: Explaining the Enigma*. New York: Wiley-Blackwell.

Garcia, Shernaz B., Anita Mendez Perez, and Alba A. Ortiz. 2000. "Mexican American Mothers' Beliefs about Disabilities: Implications for Early Childhood Intervention." *Remedial and Special Education* 21 (2):90–120.

Geertz, Hildred. 1961. *The Javanese Family: A Study of Kinship and Socialization*. New York: Free Press of Glencoe.

———. 1968. "*Latah* in Java: A Theoretical Paradox." *Indonesia* 5:93–104.

Glicksman, Eve. 2012. "Catching Autism Earlier." *APA Monitor* 23 (9):57–60.

Goddard, Cliff. 2001. "*Sabar, Ikhlas, Setia*: Patient, Sincere, Loyal?" *Journal of Pragmatics* 3:653–81.

Goldstein, Diane. 2004. *Once Upon a Virus: AIDS Legends and Vernacular Risk Perception*. Logan: Utah State University Press.

Good, Byron J., Subandi, and Mary-Jo DelVecchio Good. 2008. "The Subject of Mental Illness: Psychosis, Mad Violence, and Subjectivity in Indonesia." In *Subjectivity: Ethnographic Investigations*, ed. Joao Beihl, Byron J. Good, and Arthur Kleinman, 243–72. Berkeley: University of California Press.

Grinker, Roy Richard. 2007. *Unstrange Minds: Remapping the World of Autism*. New York: Basic Books.

Grinker, Roy Richard, and Kyungjin Cho. 2013. "Border Children: Interpreting Autism Spectrum Disorder in South Korea." *Ethos* 41 (1):46–74.

Helman, Cecil G. 1987. "Heart Disease and the Cultural Construction of Time: The Type A Behavior Pattern as a Western Culture–Bound Syndrome." *Social Science & Medicine* 25 (9):969–79.

Hoffman, Diane M. 2013. "Power Struggles: The Paradoxes of Emotion and Control among Child-Centered Mothers in the Privileged United States." *Ethos* 41 (1):75–97.

Hufford, David J. 1997. "Integrating Complementary and Alternative Medicine into Conventional Medical Practice." *Alternative Therapies in Health and Medicine* 3 (3):81–83.

———. 1998. "Folklore Studies Applied to Health." *Journal of Folklore Research* 35 (3):295–313.

Ingstad, Benedicte, and Susan Reynolds Whyte. 1995. *Disability and Culture*. Berkeley: University of California Press.

Jegatheesan, Brinda, Peggy J. Miller, and Susan A. Fowler. 2010. "Autism from a Religious Perspective: A Study of Parental Beliefs in South Asian Muslim Immigrant Families." *Focus on Autism and Other Developmental Disabilities* 25 (2):98–109.

Jones, Michael Owen. 2007. "Food Choice, Symbolism, and Identity: Bread and Butter Issues for Folkloristics and Nutrition Studies." *Journal of American Folklore* 120 (476):129–77.

Jones, Michael Owen, Patrick Polk, Ysamur Flores-Pena, and Roberta Evanchuk. 2001. "Invisible Hospitals: Botanicas in Ethnic Health Care." In *Healing Logics: Culture and Medicine in Modern Health Belief Systems*, ed. Erika Brady, 39–87. Logan: Utah State University Press.

Kanner, Leo. 1943. "Autistic Disturbances of Affective Contact." *Nervous Child* 2 (3):217–50.

Kapp, Steven. 2011. "Navajo and Autism: The Beauty of Harmony." *Disability & Society* 26 (5):583–95.

Keeler, Ward. 1983. "Shame and Stage Fright in Java." *Ethos* 11 (3):152–65.

———. 1987. *Javanese Shadow Plays, Javanese Selves*. Princeton, NJ: Princeton University Press.

Keller, Heidi. 2007. *Cultures of Infancy*. Mahwah, NJ: Lawrence Erlbaum Associates.

Khisbiyah, Yayah. 2004. *Pendidikan Apresiasi Seni: Wacana dan Praktik Untuk Toleransi Pluralism Budaya*. Surakarta, Indonesia: Pusat Studi Budaya dan Perubahan Sosial.

Kim, Hyun Uk. 2012. "Autism across Cultures: Rethinking Autism." *Disability & Society* 27 (4):535–45.

Kitta, Andrea. 2012. *Vaccinations and Public Concern in History: Legend, Rumor, and Risk Perception*. Routledge Studies in the History of Science, Technology, and Medicine. New York: Routledge.

Knapp, Julie, and Caroline Turnbull. 2014. *A Complete ABA Curriculum*. London: Jessica Kingsley.

Kodrat, Harsono. 1982. *Gending-gending Karawitan Jawa Lengkap Slendro Pelog*. Jakarta, Indonesia: Balai Pustaka.

Koen, Benjamin, ed. 2008. *The Oxford Handbook of Medical Ethnomusicology*. Oxford: Oxford University Press.

Lappe, Martine. 2013. "Anticipating Autism: Bodies of Science and Questions of Cause in the Post-genomic Era." Paper presented at the Science, Technology, and Society Series, Los Angeles, California, March 13.

Leask, J., A. Leask, and N. Silove. 2005. "Evidence for Autism in Folklore?" *Archive of Diseases in Childhood* 90 (3):271.

Levy, Susan E., David S. Mandell, Stephanie Merhar, Richard F. Ittenbach, and Jennifer A. Pinto-Marten. 2003. "Use of Complementary and Alternative Medicine among Children Recently Diagnosed with Autistic Spectrum Disorder." *Journal of Developmental & Behavioral Pediatrics* 24 (6):418–23.

Lovas, Ivar O. 1987. "Behavioral Treatment and Normal Educational and Intellectual Functioning in Young Autistic Adults." *Journal of Consulting and Clinical Psychology* 55 (1):3–9.

MacDonald, Raymond A. R., P. J. O'Donnell, and John B. Davies. 1999. "An Empirical Investigation into the Effects of Structured Music Workshops for Individuals with Intellectual Disabilities." *Journal of Applied Research in Intellectual Disabilities* 12 (3):225–40.

Matson, Johnny L., and Mathew J. Konst. 2013. "What Is the Evidence for Long-term Effects of Early Autism Interventions?" *Research in Autism Spectrum Disorders* 7 (3):475–79.

McIntosh, Jonathan. 2005. "Playing with Teaching Techniques: Gamelan as a Learning Tool amongst Children with Learning Impairments in Northern Ireland." *Anthropology in Action* 12 (2):12–27.

Mulder, Nels. 1994. *Inside Indonesian Society: Cultural Change in Java*. Singapore: Pepin Press.

Murray, Stuart. 2010. *Autism*. New York: Routledge.

Myers, Scott M., and Chris Plauche Johnson. 2007. "Management of Children with Autism Spectrum Disorders." *American Academy of Pediatrics* 120 (5):1162–82.

Nadesan, Majia Homer. 2005. *Constructing Autism: Unraveling the "Truth" and Understanding the Social*. New York: Routledge.

O'Connor, Bonnie B. 1995. *Healing Traditions: Alternative Medicine and the Health Professions*. Philadelphia: University of Pennsylvania Press.

O'Connor, Bonnie B., and David J. Hufford. 2001. "Understanding Folk Medicine." In *Healing Logics: Culture and Medicine in Modern Health Belief Systems*, ed. Erika Brady, 13–35. Logan: Utah State University Press.

Ohta, Masataka, Yoko Nagai, Hitoshi Hara, and Masami Sasaki. 1987. "Parental Perception of Behavioral Symptoms in Japanese Autistic Children." *Journal of Autism and Developmental Disorders* 17 (4):549–63.

Prijosusilo, Bramantyo. 2011. "Indonesia Needs the Harmony of the Gamelan." *Jakarta Globe* (Indonesia). February 22.

Rothbaum, Fred, Martha Pott, Hiroshi Azuma, Kazuo Miyake, and John Weisz. 2000. "The Development of Close Relationships in Japan and the United States: Paths of Symbiotic Harmony and Generative Tension." *Child Development* 71 (5):1121–42.

Sanger, Annette, and James Kippen. 1987. "Applied Ethnomusicology: The Use of Balinese Gamelan in Recreational and Educational Music Therapy." *British Journal of Music Education* 4 (1):5–16.

Santino, Jack. 1985. "On the Nature of Healing as a Folk Event." *Western Folklore* 44 (3):153–67.

Sarasvati. 2004. *Meniti Pelangi: Perjalanan Seorang Ibu yang Tak Kenal Menyerah Dalam Membimbing Putranya Keluar dari Belenggu ADHD dan Autisme*. Jakarta, Indonesia: Elex Media Komputindo.

Shaked, Michal, and Yoram Bilu. 2006. "Grappling with Affliction: Autism in the Jewish Ultra-orthodox Community in Israel." *Culture, Medicine, and Psychiatry* 30 (1):1–27.

Shuman, Amy. 2011. "On the Verge: Phenomenology and Empathic Unsettlement." *Journal of American Folklore* 124 (493):147–74.

———. 2013. "Rethinking Communicative Competence and an Argument for the Significance of Disability Studies in Folklore." Paper presented at the Annual Meeting of the American Folklore Society, Providence, RI, October 16–19.

Skinner, Deborah, and Thomas Weisner. 2007. "Sociocultural Studies of Families of Children with Intellectual Disabilities." *Mental Retardation and Developmental Disabilities Research Reviews* 13:302–12.

Subandi. 2009. "Indigenous Processes of Recovery from Psychosis in Java." Paper presented at the Workshop on Mental Health System Development for the Severe Mental Illness in Asian Countries, Taipei, Taiwan, November 3–12.

———. 2011. "Family Expressed Emotion in a Javanese Cultural Context." *Culture, Medicine and Psychiatry* 35 (3):331–46.

Susteya, W. 2007. *Dhalang, Wayang, dan Gamelan.* Yogyakarta, Indonesia: Narasi.

Sutarto, Ayu. 2006. "Becoming a True Javanese: A Javanese View of Attempts at Javanisation." *Indonesia and the Malay World* 34 (98):39–53.

Toelken, Barre. 2001. "The Hozho Factor: The Logic of Navajo Healing." In *Healing Logics: Culture and Medicine in Modern Health Belief Systems,* ed. Erika Brady, 197–208. Logan: Utah State University Press.

Tucker, Annie. 2013. "The Interpretation and Treatment of Autism in Javanese Indonesia." PhD diss., University of California, Los Angeles.

Vickers, Adrian. 2005. *A History of Modern Indonesia.* Cambridge: Cambridge University Press.

Weisner, Thomas S. 1996. "Why Ethnography Should Be the Most Important Method in the Study of Human Development." In *Ethnography and Human Development: Context and Meaning in Social Inquiry,* ed. Richard Jessor, Anne Colby, and Richard A. Schweder, 305–25. Chicago: University of Chicago Press.

Wendell, Susan. 2000. *The Rejected Body: Feminist Philosophical Reflections on Disability.* New York: Routledge.

White, John F. 2003. "Intestinal Pathophysiology in Autism." *Experimental Biology and Medicine* 228 (6):639–49.

Woodward, Mark R. 1985. "Healing and Morality: A Javanese Example." *Social Science & Medicine* 21 (9):1007–21.

CHAPTER SIX

"Heal Thyself": Holistic Women Healers in Middle America

—Elaine J. Lawless

The night before I was to leave town on a European trip, I went to the urgent care unit at my university hospital around 7:00 pm for acute sciatic pain in my left leg. I was the only patient in the waiting room. I was called in right away, and the doctor came in—a soft-spoken, calm white woman who appeared to be about fifty years old. Her slightly graying hair fell loosely down her back. She asked me to lie down on the table while she manipulated my hip joint to ascertain why I was in such pain. After only a few minutes of asking questions and probing here and there, she stepped back a bit, looked at me curiously and asked if I would mind if she performed some "alternative healing" on me. I suppose that I was too shocked to say "no," so I found myself telling her I would actually appreciate it. I was eager to try anything. She moved, then, to the end of the table and stood behind my head, gently holding my skull in the palms of her hands. She slowly and carefully manipulated my head, cradling it back, encouraging me to release it fully into her hands, telling me to trust her to move it as she wished. I tried to comply. She performed several other gentle manipulations under my ribs and chest, at my hips, and held my feet for quite some time about twelve inches in the air while standing at the foot of the table. Then, moving more quickly, she walked around my body, moving her hands lightly just above my body as though she was "feeling" the air around me, murmuring softly under her breath, indicating for me where she felt "hot spots."

Finally, with quick, brisk movements, she began to scoop the air from above various sections of my body and dump that air into the sink in the corner of the room. She did this several times, back and forth from the table to the sink. When she stopped these movements, she stood over me with her hands above my hip and told me she thought I would now be able to walk without too much difficultly. A bit stunned, I got off the table and staggered out the door, drove home, and left the next morning for my European trip.

Now, many years later, I cannot actually say if what happened in that urgent care clinic at the University Hospital cured the pain in my leg. I can, however, say that I got on the plane the next morning, walked a great deal over the next ten days, and cannot recall enduring any pain. Perhaps my ability to get up the next morning and leave Missouri as scheduled was simply my own determination, but I do in fact know the healing moment in the urgent care clinic late that night had a profound effect on me far beyond any "healing" that might have happened. As a folklorist interested in women's healing practices, I was more than a little surprised that a medical doctor had asked if she could do "alternative healing" on me in a university hospital room. Little did she know I was a woman ripe for such an experience, an academic who has spent a career reading and writing about belief and religious practice. I have often wondered how she could have known that I would be open to her alternative healing methods rather than report her to the authorities. Eventually, someone actually did report her activities, and she was eventually asked to leave the hospital, which made it quite difficult for me to relocate her when I wanted to write about her as a "healer."[1]

At the time I first met her, I had no idea this physician was part of a local "healing community" of women who regularly meet, share knowledge, and practice various healing modalities in the small academic town where I live. In addition to learning from each other on a regular basis, they also are exposed to and learn new healing practices offered by healers who occasionally visit from other areas, so mouth-to-mouth and hand-to-hand learning about healing takes place all the time. Some of the women in this group regularly treat clients in healing sessions in clinics, while others offer it along with massage therapy in their homes. They all claim a holistic approach to healing that includes attention to complex understandings of how mind, body, and spirit work in conjunction for healing the human body. This approach guides their daily lives as well as their healing practices.

In the cold, poorly-lit physical therapy labs in the basement of an older university building, the healing women meet to teach each other, to "work" on each other, to do the practice, and share healing beliefs and stories. People who come to these women healers for "healing" come during and after their regular biomedical treatments, seeking a practice that is not available elsewhere—they seek touch, understanding, intimacy, spiritual connection, and support for their own belief that they will benefit from seeking healing in addition to their biomedical patient care. I would agree with Bonnie O'Connor that these complementary systems of belief are not fragmented or disconnected but, rather, constitute an "organized coherent system of thought" about the complexity and the integration of the mind and the body, the spirit, and the soul (1995:22). But the terms included in "complementary systems of belief" carry baggage that makes it difficult to do this research and give it fair scholarly treatment.

Learning about this group and coming to an understanding of their practices has taken many years. In the meantime, in what I initially perceived as completely unrelated activities, I have been busy teaching, writing, taking trips, and exploring new experiences that have felt to me both like ethnographic journeys and New Age spirituality adventures. Until now, trying to write about how these journeys happened, and how they are actually connected to the women healers, has made as little sense as writing about the encounter in the hospital urgent care unit. Now I recognize how these seemingly different paths are connected in many powerful ways. This essay seeks to write my own experiences with a group of Midwestern healing women and my own participation in their healing efforts—a journey that has enabled me to connect my academic and personal work in meaningful ways. My work in this area has been enhanced by Eric Lassiter's (2001) work on collaborative ethnography. In his article, Lassiter takes my own notion of reciprocal ethnography, which insists that we include the participants of our studies in the writing of the research and suggests that we need to not only read over the shoulders of our participants, but also read alongside them. I would like to take Lassiter's point one step further and argue that in our work, we need to "read with" our participants. By this I mean we step into the ethnography as participants. I realize there are many ethnographies that depend upon on the ethnographer going native and others that are critical of this full immersion. In this case, I was actually required to participate in the healing activities in ways I had never been expected to participate in my other ethnographic research projects. By accepting the terms of my research and participation, I must also accept my own participation in the ethnographic journey. By examining what happened to me in this project, I am in a position to suggest that in our work we travel with our participants in ways that go beyond both reflexive and reciprocal ethnography.

Both Ruth Behar and Luice Giudice argue for ethnographic vulnerability that "challenge[s] the 'ethnological imagination' to en-vision a rare border crossing between ethnography and spiritual direction" (Behar 1996:174) and to consider the ways in which "deep listening may in effect be considered a form of spiritual practice" (Giudice 2007:28). Their words resonate with me, particularly as each of these ethnographers talk about their own spiritual paths and how those paths intersect with their academic paths. As I slowly became aware of the many intersections of ethnography and spirituality at the core of my own life, my research, and advocacy, I am surprised that it took so long to recognize and articulate the intimate connections between and among such powerful presences in my life and my research.

For years, I have studied and written books about clergywomen, both Pentecostal and mainline denominational pastors in the Midwest (Lawless 1988a, 1988b, 1993, 1996). Belief, religion, and how people make meaning spiritually are issues I find important to study. As sometimes happens, a number of the women I studied for those earlier publications have become my dear friends over time. Following the publication of my books about the clergywomen and the successful use of reciprocal ethnography, where I invited the participants to read what I was writing about them and to help me frame what the books included, I began to travel with some of my collaborators to conferences and events that offered insights into issues of spirituality, healing, and clergywomen's rights.

Years before, I had denounced all my ties to the fundamentalist Christian religion in which I had been raised. In my research, I had never felt inclined to join any of the faith communities of the clergywomen I was researching. Over my years of participatory study with them, they seemed to be content to have me join them in these spiritual retreats. Attending the conferences, seminars, and lectures felt too natural to be "only" fieldwork, and I was diligent with my journaling throughout all these trips, conferences, and spiritual encounters. As it happens, the more I tried to write about these spiritual journeys, the more difficult it became to write about "them" (the other women) and "us" (the traveling seekers, which both did and did not include me). Even though I do not self-identify as a religious person, I do recognize and honor the power of the spiritual, and I felt that traveling with the women I was writing about would enhance my understanding of their faith and their spirituality. It took me longer to acknowledge that some of this spiritual work was for me, personally, as well. As we confided in each other over the course of several years, "they" began to also articulate how they felt I had become one of "them," yet I did not completely understand why.

Certainly, the women I have come to know through my research recognize me as someone who respects spirituality; perhaps, more to the point, they also see me as possessing a need for spirituality, a searcher or seeker, someone with an equal need. They view me as a "re-searcher," which gives me legitimacy within their group. As long as I am a re-searcher who genuinely wants to learn more about spirituality, the lines between ethnographer and active participant have become blurred; ethnography and personal memoir both find their way into my writing. Certainly, my role as researcher of the spiritual results in part from my discomfort with the purely academic life I lead. I have always felt there ought to be something more to life than what the academic world has to offer—a world where open discussion of the soul, the spiritual, or the possibilities of personal transformation are mostly forbidden, unless, of course, we are discussing Keats, Wordsworth, or, perhaps, William James. Personal spiritual quests in the English Department are pretty much available only to the poets. Thus, my life during these years of journeys and journaling, research, writing, and teaching represent a life of bifurcation. At the university I am a professor; on the spiritual journeys, I am a researcher, but also a friend and a seeker, someone willing to learn with my new friends and colleagues. Most of the time with the women I study, I have felt included, welcomed, and even loved—feelings that I have rarely encountered on the university campus. In essence, however, I have become like Ruth Behar's "vulnerable observer" in that I felt the lines of distinction fall away as personal and ethnographic writing facilitate exchanges which become autoethnographic and autobiography that become more ethnographic (Behar 1996:19). The "they" and the "we" are not readily available to me anymore as I write about the women in this study—a group of women that now includes me.

How did the healing group in the town in which I reside come to intersect with the group of spiritual travelers I have come to know over the past several years? I can begin to make the connection in this way: the group of women who traveled to France together included clergywomen, church leaders, laywomen, artists, mothers, sisters, friends, and me. We are all well-educated, professional women who had the means to travel in France for nearly two weeks, visiting museums and cathedrals, universities and retreat centers, seeking evidence of historical and religious iconography of the "feminine divine." My work as a scholar interested in belief and religious practice melded nicely with the intentions of these traveling women. I know the mythology, and I recognized the characters in the various icons we studied in the dusty lower levels of museums, eager to hear the stories of the Black Madonna told in the crypts of ancient cathedrals. Like some of the other women on the trip, I had not actively searched for evidence of the "divine feminine." We all had to find ways to incorporate this new knowledge and understanding within our own spiritual perceptions. For me, it was a positive experience that helped me articulate where some of my anger toward religion, especially southern Baptist fundamentalist religion, originated. At a young age, I noticed the lack of female voices in male dominated God-talk, the hymns, the hellfire and brimstone preaching, as well as the iconography that basically only included biblical depictions of God and His Son. Actually *seeing* female images of the divine alongside male images of the divine, the manifestation of the divine within the human, in Mary as the Madonna not inferior to God and Christ, helped me breathe a little easier. I longed for the wisdom and power of Sophia,[2] and we seemed to find her on those travels.

Lucky for us, our travels in France culminated with permission to walk the labyrinth at Chartres Cathedral. It took us three days to convince the rector to remove all the folding chairs from the labyrinth,[3] but late one night when no one else was on the grounds, he complied and allowed us to walk the labyrinth in the shadows of the awe-inspiring walls and tapestries of Chartres Cathedral, flickering in the soft light of a thousand votive candles. Later, we shared the stories of the connections between the Virgin, the labyrinth, the Rose windows, and the architecture of the cathedral itself. The experience was overwhelmingly powerful, lasting, and intensely satisfying. I learned a great deal on that trip, but perhaps most important for me personally was the discovery of the spiritual connections between women on a similar path.

Some of us continued our work studying labyrinths the following year in San Francisco with the Reverend Lauren Artress, one of the priests at Grace Cathedral at that time, who installed two Chartres labyrinth replicas (one inside the sanctuary, one outside on the grounds) at the very peak of Nob Hill, where San Francisco lies at one's feet as far as you can see before the water of the ocean expands the view to the horizon. I was ready to study the labyrinth—the various forms of the meditative labyrinth walk, how different labyrinths could be made with different materials; of the earth, upon the earth, carved out of the earth. For the first time, my research actually helped me slow down, because regularly walking different labyrinths takes time and encourages contemplation. As with folklorist Maida Owens, my journaling about walking the labyrinth and spiritual practice took a different turn.[4]

Eventually, a clergywoman from my various research projects suggested the two of us develop a weekend workshop in Kansas City to explore images of the feminine divine in the Nelson-Atkins Museum and other local spiritual retreats, including one that had a labyrinth we could walk together as a group. Incidentally, or not, several of the women who signed up for our trip to Kansas City were members of the women's healing group in Columbia—the same group that included the female doctor I first met in the University Emergency Care Unit. The overlapping interests were significant; the language on this trip was about holistic understandings of not only the feminine divine, but also how the divine manifests within each person, including, and in this context especially, how *women need to take responsibility for their own healing.*

Eventually, our labyrinth work took some of us to New Mexico and South Africa and finally back to Columbia, Missouri. Here, the women healers and clergywomen worked for months with a local hospital to build an outdoor, wheelchair accessible, Chartres-inspired healing labyrinth, blessed both day and night by a soaring life-sized sculpture of an eagle in flight, designed and created by one of our local artist friends.

The night of the dedication of the Columbia labyrinth, my clergywoman friend and traveling companion led the prayer service. Also at the dedication were several women I did not know, but soon I learned they were nearly all long-standing participants in the local group of women healers who practice energy work together; they were equally delighted to see the healing labyrinth now in place. After the dedication, we stood around the edges of the labyrinth in the twilight, and the women began to talk about their healing work and why the labyrinth was such a blessing and an important spiritual addition to our community. One of the women had been working for years to get this labyrinth built, saving every dollar she earned in her healing ministry to help pay the labyrinth artist. Inspired, I asked if I could visit her and learn more about her energy work. She was open, inviting, and eager to share what she knew. She told me I could come see her the following day at her home and she would teach me the practice. And then she invited me to attend the twice-monthly meetings of the healing group. There is no more inspired moment in an ethnographer's research life than an invitation such as this! I knew then that I would write about this group of healers; little did I realize how long it would take to make the connections I needed to make about healing, belief, and spirituality.

Months later, when I attended a gathering of these healing women, to my great delight the very doctor who had done the alternative healing work on me at the university hospital urgent care unit came through the door, arriving late. The others greeted her as a beloved member who had been absent for some time. I was astonished. I had found her again, and the pieces of this ethnographic puzzle began to connect in ways not yet revealed to me but were certainly promising.

In 2008, when I first interviewed her, I told her I had been looking for her ever since that night at the hospital, but my searching had always hit a dead end. The hospital refused to tell me where she was practicing or tell me what had happened to her, which made me curious, if not suspicious. Sometimes I wondered if I had dreamed the strange encounter. "And I have tried to find *you*," she said, to my amazement. "I mean, I've wondered and wondered how your trip went and how your leg was. That night, I felt you were someone I could trust with these new therapies." In our interview, she continued:

> I was working in Urgent Care [and] there were lots of really good opportunities to use it [her healing powers], but the "powers that be" [the university hospital administration] were not too thrilled with it. [There] I would do the Western medicine thing first—then, I'd think, "OK, we're done [with that]—but if we've evaluated, and we've come up with the best treatment Western medicine has [and it's not working] and there's nobody waiting"—[we both laughed] then I would ask the patient "you want something a little extra?" And I would close the door and try new modalities, and, you know, there were several people that I was able to really help that way. But, there were one or two that were pretty freaked out by it, and it got me into trouble. Eventually, you know, I had to leave there.[5]

She had been asked to leave the hospital and is now in private practice, a medical practice her business card describes as "intuitive, integrative, and holistic medicine." The university hospital pretends not to know who she is and will not give any information about her current practice.

Interestingly, involvement with this group of Midwestern, white, middle-class women healers has been far more intimate than I am normally comfortable with in my field research—and this includes twenty years of working with religious groups, such as the Pentecostal believers, who often worried for my soul and felt it might be helpful for me to become a *believer*. This work has also proven to be even more difficult than the years spent in dialogue with clergywomen as I developed the notion of "reciprocal ethnography," which demands we share our academic writing with the participants in our studies. With the clergywomen, I was never urged to convert or join any of their denominations. But in this new ethnographic work with women healers, I have not been able to maintain my position as detached ethnographer, largely because this work has required more of my own participation than ever before. Overall, their insistence upon my participation has both interrupted the ethnographic project but, simultaneously, enhanced my own spiritual journey. With Ruth Behar, I note the near impossibility of writing about others without writing about ourselves:

> Writing vulnerably takes as much skill, nuance, and willingness to follow through on all the ramifications of a complicated idea as does writing invulnerably and distantly. I would say it takes yet greater skill. When an author has made herself vulnerable, the stakes are higher. (Behar 1996:13)

Behar explains vulnerable writing as writing that "breaks your heart" in that if one writes vulnerably, the reader will share in that vulnerability. She calls this "mediated autobiography," a new genre that privileges the subjective while acknowledging that self-reflexivity is not an end to itself: "How do you write subjectivity into ethnography in such a way that you can continue to call what you are doing ethnography?" (1996:7).

From the outset of my work with women healers, I was told, "Yes, you may come to our healing gatherings, but you must learn to heal if you want to come." I hedged, claiming "Well, right now, I just want to watch what you do and observe." This was not an option. Without wavering, they informed me that I could come only if I "learned the practice. It does not matter if you believe or not. Belief and practice are one. You must do the practice. It is in the doing that the healing is done. If you want to come, you must learn to do the practice." Therefore, not long after the dedication of the labyrinth, I went to see the healer who had invited me to learn from her and agreed to her methods of learning to heal. For her, the teaching of the healing process was first to practice the hands-on modalities she preferred, which involved mostly cranial-sacral energy work, talking me through what she was doing. She began with my feet, holding them in her warm hands about a foot above the table until she felt the energy in my body had reached a "still point." From there, she moved to my head and cradled it within her hands, also lifting it off the table, asking me, again, to relax within her hands and trust her hands to do the work they know so well. She quietly talked me through her methods, explaining each movement and asking me to focus on what occurred in my body at each point of her finger and hand pressure. She did this for an hour on several different occasions, noting my energy chakras and indicating where she felt the energy to be "hot," "cold," or "out of harmony." (There were many of these spots, as I recall.) Throughout her healing sessions on me, she was explaining to me what she was doing and why, as well as pointing out what I would need to do once I began healing practice on others. Weeks later, she invited another new learner to her home, and she taught us to practice the methods on each other, quietly and patiently asking us to trust that our hands could do the work if we just "did the practice."

My complicity grew. Late one night Louise brought a young girl she knew who was going into the hospital the following day for kidney surgery to the women's group in the therapy lab for healing. The girl was slight and pale, but she was calm and smiling at all of us. Louise indicated that the girl should get up onto one of the tables, motioning for all of us to gather around the girl. I remember the girl's mother was there, standing by her side, holding her left hand. Each of the women in the group, *including me*, stood at different places near the girl's body. I knew what to do by this point based on what I had been taught in the various sessions. With the other healers, I put my hands near her neck, which was the body part closest to me in the circle. All of us held our hands about four inches above the girl's body; we closed our eyes and began to "feel" the energy just below our palms and fingers. It felt natural for me to concentrate on the energy I could feel emanating from this young girl's body; without any direction from me, my hands began to gently circle counterclockwise above her neck. For a moment, I allowed my eyes to open in order to observe that all the other women were similarly drawing small circles above the girl's body, feeling the air and attempting to feel the energy emanating from her body at different points. No one said a word; there was no singing, no chanting, no spoken concerns, no prayers offered, until nearly twenty minutes had passed. Then, from the other side of the table, near the girl's left thigh, I heard the voice of Louise deliver a quiet prayer, as I remember it:

> Please be with Emma tonight and tomorrow and for as long as she needs your blessed attention. Go into that operation room with her and guide the hands of the surgeons. Help her body be strong and able to fight infections. Give her strength to trust that she can be healed. Bless our collective energy here to help her on her path toward being whole again.

We remained in our places for some moments after her words. As I opened my eyes, I could see that all the women were now touching the girl in loving ways, telling her to be brave and trust that everything would be all right. Her mother was openly weeping and thanking all of us for our healing energy. The girl's mother had asked this group of healers to pray over her daughter before she went into the hospital. The girl and her mother had not chosen this healing session as an alternative to the surgeon's knife in the local hospital, but they had desired something more than the hospital could provide. Our healing session brought the spiritual energy this woman believed would assist her daughter as she subjected herself to the hospital's care. Body, mind, and spirit coalesced in that moment; the energy in that room was more powerful than any I had ever witnessed in my life, or at least that is how I personally responded.

Later, I asked Louise about that night in the therapy lab, and she remembered it as vividly as I did. She talked about the power of the healing group: "I think that almost any healing ritual is really a matter of focusing your intention and, to the extent that the group helps you have confidence to do that—it helps you focus your intention." This was another refrain I would hear again and again, that healing is about "fixing an intention." And, for the first time during this research (or any other), she asked me what I had felt that night. I did not remember how I had answered her until I was reading my transcripts again for this essay. I had answered, "nothing I can put into words. It was just that I felt so much a part of the community there, of women—and her [the girl], and her mother. I think it was the connection, because I didn't know what I could give her. I didn't have any confidence at all. But that my hands were there with all of your hands was profound. Just profound."

I began attending and participating in the healing gatherings several years ago, but I did not interview many of the women healers until several years later. In their conversations with me, they all refer to themselves (in one way or another) as healers. Most have a story that they tell about their calling to be a healer; many talk openly about how they negotiate their healing within the biomedical institutions in which many of them work and how they do, or do not, negotiate the conflicts. Some told me stories of how they healed individual people; some talked about their own doubts but how the healing process always reinserts itself into their lives. Many of these women attribute their abilities to God or Spirit (the Chi) and claim only to be a conduit for divine healing powers that are already available to the patient. All of them see themselves as testaments to their own faith: they live what they believe. This is not a new concept; most believers of any faith might say the same thing. Beth Hathaway, a tai chi teacher and healer, talked openly with me about how radically her life had changed. Before, as a busy wife and mother of three, she was always in a flurry, running around town, frazzled, with many medical conditions and taking many drug prescriptions. Then she began to take tai chi and yoga; she took up meditation, learned various healing practices first by experiencing them for herself, then seeking the training to help others heal physically, emotionally, and spiritually. "I live what I teach," she says. "People who know me see the difference. They ask me what I am doing differently now. They notice that I am 'not sick, harried, a mess [she laughs].'" "So, first, they see the effects of the practice in my life, then they come to me for guidance and for healing." But "healing," she warns me, "does not necessarily mean being 'cured.'" I nod. I have heard this many times before. "Healing is a journey; healing means being in control of your breath, letting your body move, letting go. And, if you can do that, you heal yourself. The pain will lessen. You will heal."[6]

Louise, my elusive medical doctor gone rogue, spent hours with me sharing her story about her desire to be a nurse, but how she went to medical school instead at the insistence of her father. Even as a child, she had felt a pull to heal. She told me about an experience that happened while she was at a church camp:

> But I woke up in the middle of the night so I knew there was a reason. I was like: What is it God? Here I am! And, my top bunk was right by this window

that was about that big [opens her hands long and wide], and I looked out the window and the moon was full. I thought, oh, how sweet, you woke me up to look at the moon. I was just admiring it and saying "thank you," and I laid back on my bed and put my hands up, and, I felt like God was telling me he wanted to bless my hands and I was like: "Well, thank you!" you know, "I don't know what that's for but I promise I'll quit complaining about how big and manly my hands look and learn to heal" [she laughed].

I feel like you're the perfect person for me to tell this story to [Louise says to me] because my beginning, my whole journey in life, it has been spiritual, you know, a seeking. Even as a young child, I have felt that mystical connection. . . . But the more, the longer I got into medicine the more I wondered if this was really what I really wanted. What I wanted to do is help people heal spiritually. [Being a doctor] is sort of like being a car mechanic, pretty superficial. But the underlying miracle of the body is something that comes from the *self*. What really would send me home singing was if once every four or six months, the medical encounter would end up with me being able to help someone untie one of those emotional knots. And I would see that person go out feeling more free psychologically or emotionally, and I would feel like, ok, now I love my work!

Louise began to learn different spiritual modalities that might connect with her medical practice. She was having fun, she told me, "I had some fabulous experiences—some of them disorienting and some were just really tickling and fun. So, from then on I kept looking for people to try it on, you know. And it was round that time when I ran into you—in urgent care."[7]

Louise is not the only medical professional to leave the biomedical world to practice their passion. Helen Gallagher held a PhD in Occupational Therapy and was a clinical assistant professor at the university where I taught at the time of my interview with her. She told me about her long journey from a community college program to medical school and finally the PhD as a clinical researcher, but her heart, she told me, wasn't in it:

It's a delicate balance. The university could use all of your energy in the Biomedical model and certainly that's where we put a lot of our resources and our faith. But I also put some of my energy and resources, and *a lot of my faith* in what I call just simple, practical healing methods. We say the problem is not enough money or not enough training, but, in fact, we're not paying attention to the things that make people *heal*, and it can be as simple as having sunlight coming into your room when you are sick. Or, it can be as simple as paying attention to your breathing, listening to your own body and listening to what it is trying to tell you. In the biomedical model, we have wonderful tools, we have a blizzard of information, but we don't often get training in how to *listen* and apply what we hear or learn appropriately.

I think sometimes we barrage people with tests, with therapies, speech therapy, occupational therapy, physical therapy, and you need to see a psychologist, and take all these medications and pretty soon it's just overwhelming. And, in the process, we often lose touch with the human contact that is healing, the *hands-on aspect*. With children; it was the energy and the movement. I began to take and then teach tai chi and yoga, and that's what fed my spirit, you know. It helped me acknowledge balance. It helped me stay focused and meditative and yet stay healthy.

So, when I went into OT [occupational therapy], I had this idea that I would be able to do "hands-on" therapy with people and I would have a legitimate credential to do that. So that I would build some trust with people and get to say "come, lay on my table." But some people were, you know, some are still a little suspicious of that.[8]

Helen explained how all her degrees and credentials did not provide ways for her to do the work she really wanted to do, things that would support healing. She thought a great deal about the role of the hands in healing, "not just physically, but through the energy and the emotional, the relationship when you help a person relax into a place where their body heals itself." "That," she claims, "is the model that holds true for me." She began to quietly complete a four-year course in Chicago in Feldenkrais, another "awareness through movement" healing modality program, stealing time from her research at the university, staying up all night to grade her students' papers. Six weeks after my interview with her, she quit her position at the university to open her own Feldenkrais space with another local body awareness healer. Her website features her photo, a smiling middle-aged woman in a fluid body posture. The text reads:

Healing movement can change not only the way we move, but the way we think and feel as well. I teach group classes and individual sessions as a certified tai chi instructor and as a certified Feldenkrais practitioner. After retiring from my occupational therapy career I wanted to devote my energies to healing practices that help people prevent illness and maintain their health.

Obviously, this website caption does not tell the whole story, but it offers what she sees as a satisfying turn in her journey. She looks very happy in the photo.

One of the women who accompanied us to Kansas City in search of the "feminine divine" is a local massage therapist, energy worker, and teacher of many different body/mind/spirit modalities. Marian Copeland manages her own private therapy sessions, and she also helps the local medical units integrate alternative and complementary therapies into their protocol. Her own enthusiasm for energy work, both on our trips and our meditative labyrinth walks was obvious. Like the other practitioners, she strives to "live what she teaches, believes, and practices." At sixty, she does not take a single prescription medication herself, rarely visits medical doctors unless absolutely necessary, and is a specimen of good health and energy, sparkling with life and love for everything on the planet. Her story paralleled many of the others. She was careful about claiming the role of "healer," although she says she does think of herself in that way. One thing she kept repeating was what others had said as well:

> Healing is not the same as curing. That word "healing" has many, many levels of meaning and connotations. What healing means to you may not be what it means to me and we may be talking about healing our toe or a bigger, more emotional heart issue. Healing is multi-leveled. Healing is not the same as "cured." I would say, in fact, that cancer has "healed" a lot of people. They may not be cured, but they are healed.[9]

For Marian, in fact, none of us are ever likely to actually be healed. However, she believes, we are all on what she calls a "healing path." How we navigate this journey depends upon how we become active participants in our own life and our own healing. When I asked her to explain if she identified as a healer, she paused for a long time to think about the answer:

> I would hope so. I mean in my heart of hearts, I hope I help people on their healing path. To be labeled as a healer is a big responsibility. But yes, I would say with the broader meaning that I hope that I help people heal in the grocery store and in all my activities. I hope that my interactions and my relationships, however brief or long they are, become a healing experience for both of us. And, it *is* a healing for the broader planet when we put that healing energy out there. I put myself into an "intention" that I want to put healing energy in every action that I do. I see a lot of pain in the world and the only way we're going to heal it is one step at a time. One relationship at a time. And it changes the energy of the planet each time, just a little bit more, just a little bit more.[10]

Louise, Beth, Helen, and Marian, as well as the other women in this group of healing women, are modest in their claims for the ability to heal others, yet all of them live what they believe.

I feel privileged to have access to this group of women dedicated to the power of hands-on healing, the power of women learning to heal together, the power of belief for healing, and the belief that practice is more important that believing it will work. They tell me they "live what they teach." By claiming they are just a conduit for a "larger power," they deflect attention from their own abilities, as women often do. Yet they also admit to being in close contact with spirit, spiritual matters and beings, energy, and life force. Whatever language they use, they believe they hold a special position as a vessel for healing energy to be transmitted from the source (of healing), through them, to the person seeking help. They see no conflict in also recognizing divine feminine power in themselves and in their clients. They tell me they can sense and feel, with only a bit of observation and touching, what is ailing a person and they then, seek to help the client dispel whatever imbalance might be present; they claim to know how to help the person on their table restore harmony in her own body. Marian said it so well: "I think, unless [clients] are open to finding their own healing potential, in a sense they're never going to be completely healed. If they expect somebody else to do it for them."[11] In this way, the healers are self-effacing; they seek no acclaim for themselves. Theirs is a calling; they are here to teach us how to heal ourselves.

Researcher Bonnie Glass-Coffin reflects upon the experiences of healing in her own work, asking "whose logic, whose experience?" (1998:13). On her website we find these words: "Bonnie Glass-Coffin, Ph.D., is a visionary and a bridge builder who believes that educating the whole person (head and heart) should be at the core of a liberal arts education. She has been inspired to build these bridges because of the transformational experiences that she has had while studying with Peruvian shamans for more than 30 years." She calls for ethnography to "learn to live with the ambiguities of empiricism" (13). As researchers, she says, "we should consider the role of experience as both science and interpretive discipline" (193). I suppose that is why women healers insist on saying, "If you practice, it will work." Women healers offer hands-on care as constituting sincere acts of faith and well-being; the recipients of the healings believe they are being helped and healed or, like me, find themselves attracted to healing practices that reconnect body, mind, and spirit, are non-invasive, and often lead to a more balanced, holistic understanding of the body and its interaction with the modern world. Nothing about this work is dispassionate or value-neutral; in fact, the women themselves talk about the work as passionate, the kind of work that "feeds them." They fall in love with the power of healing. To close, I offer a prayer from one of the healers in the group in hopes that it appropriately connects the energies in this essay.

Following her energy work on my body, she often repeats some version of the following:

> We take a moment to offer a prayer of gratitude for the gift of healing—the healing of our hearts, our minds, our souls, our physical bodies. We say thank you.
>
>   Bless you, Elaine. Be well.

Notes

1. As with all my work, I utilized what I have coined as "reciprocal ethnography" (see Lawless 1993) by taking this essay to the women healers who are featured here. They loved reading it and came back with many suggestions that helped me phrase things better or make the article more comprehensible for the reader. For example, they were insistent that I refer to those who come to them for spiritual healing as *clients*, not patients. Only Dr. Dennis would be comfortable with the use of the word *patient*. I want to thank them all collectively even though they still do not wish for me to use their real or full names, which in itself perhaps says something unfortunate about the world of alternative healing by spiritual women.

2. A quick Google search reveals that "Sophia" in Greek translates as "Wisdom" and has been utilized as such throughout history, philosophy, and religion(s), often equated with the feminine aspect of the trinity.

3. The Chartres labyrinth is regularly covered with chairs except for Wednesdays, when visitors can walk the labyrinth. Walking the labyrinth has long been part of spiritual practice around the world. See Artress (2006).

4. See Owens (2009) for a good discussion of walking the labyrinth from a folklorist's point of view.

5. Author interview with Louise Dennis, Columbia, MO, October 18, 2010.

6. Author interview with Beth Hathaway, Columbia, MO, April 29, 2008.

7. Author interview with Louise Dennis, Columbia, MO, March 27, 2008.

8. Author interview with Helen Gallagher, Columbia, MO, March 27, 2008.

9. Author interview with Marian Copeland, Columbia, MO, April 19, 2009.

10. Ibid.

11. Author interview with Marian Copeland, Columbia, MO, April 29, 2008.

References

Achterberg, Jeanne. 1991. *Woman as Healer*. Boston: Shambhala.

Albanese, Catherine L. 2007. *A Republic of Mind and Spirit: A Cultural History of American Metaphysical Religion*. New Haven, CT: Yale University Press.

Artress, Lauren. 2006. *Walking a Sacred Path: Rediscovering the Labyrinth as a Spiritual Practice*. San Francisco: Riverhead Trade.

Badaracco, Claire Hoertz. 2007. *Prescribing Faith: Medicine, Media, and Religion in American Culture*. Waco, TX: Baylor University Press.

Behar, Ruth. 1996. *The Vulnerable Observer: Anthropology That Breaks Your Heart*. Boston: Beacon Press.

Bourdillon, Hilary. 1988. *Women as Healers: A History of Women and Medicine*. Cambridge: Cambridge University Press.

Brady, Erika, ed. 2001. *Healing Logics: Culture and Medicine in Modern Health Belief Systems*. Logan: Utah State University Press.

Brooke, Elisabeth. 1995. *Women Healers: Portraits of Herbalists, Physicians, and Midwives*. Rochester, VT: Healing Arts Press.

Del Giudice, Luisa. 2007. "Ethnography as Spiritual Practice." Paper presented at the American Folklore Society/Folklore Studies Association of Canada Joint Annual Meeting, Université Laval, Québec, Canada, October 17–21, 2007.

Glass-Coffin, Bonnie. 1998. *The Gift of Life: Female Spirituality and Healing in Northern Peru*. Studies in Modern German Literature. Albuquerque: University of New Mexico Press.

Kirkland, James, Holly Matthews, C. W. Sullivan III, and Karen Baldwin, eds. 1992. *Herbal and Magical Medicine: Traditional Healing Today*. Durham, NC: Duke University Press.

Lassiter, Luke Eric. 2001. "'Reading over the Shoulders of Natives' to Reading Alongside Natives, Literally: Toward a Collaborative and Reciprocal Ethnography." *Journal of Anthropological Research* 57 (2):137–49.

Lawless, Elaine. 1988a. *God's Peculiar People: Women's Voices and Folk Tradition in a Pentecostal Church*. Lexington: University Press of Kentucky.

———. 1988b. *Handmaidens of the Lord: Women Preachers and Traditional Religion*. Philadelphia: University of Pennsylvania Press and the Publications of the American Folklore Society, New Series.

———. 1993. *Holy Women, Wholly Women: Sharing Ministries through Life Stories and Reciprocal Ethnography*. Philadelphia: University of Pennsylvania Press and the Publications of the American Folklore Society, New Series.

———. 1996. *Women Preaching Revolution: Calling for Connection in a Disconnected Time*. Philadelphia: University of Pennsylvania Press.

———. 2001. *Women Escaping Violence: Empowerment through Narrative*. Columbia: University of Missouri Press.

O'Connor, Bonnie Blair. 1995. *Healing Traditions: Alternative Medicine and the Health Professions*. Philadelphia: University of Pennsylvania Press.

Ruether, Rosemary Radford, ed. 1996. *Women Healing Earth: Third World Women on Ecology, Feminism, and Religion*. New York: Orbis Books.

Visweswaran, Kamala. 1994. *Fictions of Feminist Ethnography*. Minneapolis: University of Minnesota Press.

PART THREE

The Performance of Mental Illness, Stigma, and Trauma

CHAPTER SEVEN

Deranged Psychopaths and Victims Who Go Insane: Visibility and Invisibility in the Depiction of Mental Health and Illness in Contemporary Legend

—Diane E. Goldstein

Some years ago, when collecting legends concerning HIV/AIDS, I became intrigued by a minor pattern that I observed in those narratives. One of the narratives that I collected extensively ended with the coda or punchline, "Welcome to the World of AIDS." The following text, collected in Newfoundland in 2000, is typical of the narrative:

> This girl needed a break and decided to go to Florida for a month or two holiday, I think. While she was there she met a man, who seemed to be . . . the man of her dreams. He had money, he treated her like gold and he gave her everything she wanted. She fell in love with him and . . . during the last night there they slept together. The next day he brought her to the airport for her return to St. John's. He gave her a small gift-wrapped box and told her not to open it until she got home. They . . . said goodbye and she left, hoping that they would someday be married and the gift would be an [engagement] ring. The suspense was killing her and . . . she decided to open the gift on the plane. It was a small coffin with a piece of paper saying, "Welcome to the World of AIDS." (Goldstein 2004:101)

In this (at that time) popular story, a woman or a man meets someone, has sex with that person, and receives a gift with the "welcome" message hidden inside or discovers the message written in lipstick or blood on the bathroom mirror. Generally, Welcome to the World of AIDS legends and their similar counterparts conclude with the message informing the man or woman that he or she may have been infected with the virus.[1] I would estimate that 30 percent of the eight hundred versions I collected simply ended, much like the version offered above, with the tag line and no further elaboration. Another 30 percent or so ended with the protagonist testing HIV positive. Of the remaining 40 percent, about half indicated that the individual died a day or two later, which is in itself interesting for what it might say about general knowledge of the disease's progression. But the most intriguing part was the remaining 20 percent of the narratives. In these stories, a different coda follows the young woman receiving the message. The woman, finding out that her new true love has infected her with HIV, "goes crazy." In some of these stories, the narrator indicated, "She saw the note and that was it, she lost it. They had to cart her away." Others said, "She read the message and she was never the same again. She's in the Waterford Hospital now." The majority of the narratives simply noted her collapse, indicating, as did one narrator, "She went crazy, right then and there, absolutely mad."

What intrigued me about these stories was the suggestion that the loss of one's sanity or "going crazy," as the narrators put it, was an equivalent horror or perhaps even a superior horror, to a potentially terminal illness. I felt as I read these stories that their message was that the loss of one's sanity was, in fact, a fate worse than death.[2] These stories stayed in the back of my mind for a long time, but after a while I began to notice the insanity coda cropping up occasionally in a variety of other contemporary legends—all of them horror stories, and in each case the normal climax, the unspeakable horror of the boyfriend's death[3] or the castrated boy,[4] is followed by one further horror, the girlfriend or the boy's mother going crazy.

This is not to say that the insanity coda is widespread, and in fact, description of any aftermath or set of consequences resulting from legendary events is relatively rare. Gary Alan Fine (1992) notes in his study of the Kentucky Fried Rat legend that only 13 percent of the narratives describe the harmful effects of the legend's complicating action. The example he gives of those that do mention the aftermath of the events, however, looks surprisingly familiar:

> My sister told me that her friend told her that a lady went to Kentucky Fried Chicken. She was out in the car eating it and noticed that one of the pieces tasted funny. She looked and it had a tail. Then she looked again and saw it had eyes and was a rat. She threw up and went crazy and is in the State [Mental] hospital in Kalamazoo. She won't eat any food. (Fine 1992:130–31)

A survey of contemporary legends from Memorial University's Folklore and Language Archives and the Folklore Archives of Utah State University, combined with published sources and my own field collections, suggested that the insanity coda is limited but not uncommon. The specific examples, however, are instructive. The protagonist who goes spontaneously, quietly, and completely mad in the narratives is always a woman. Thinking about other depictions of mental illness in legend fleshed out this observation, adding dimension to the few short lines provided by the brief description of legendary aftermath.

Certainly, insanity is no stranger to legend topics. Numerous contemporary legends involve the psychopathic actions of what folklorist Michael Goss has called the "urban maniac." As Goss notes, these legends use transient, unpredictable, and totally irrational psychopaths as their theme and make all the gore, carnage, and cruelty credible by engaging our preconceptions about "psychopaths and other dangers" (1990:95). Goss goes on to say, "While never inviting us to question whether such maniacs exist outside of fiction (and by implying that they certainly do!), much of the appeal of these stories lies in their gross entertainment value . . . but nevertheless, they still encapsulate certain values and act as cautionary tales" (95).

I would like to explore the portrayal of mental illness in contemporary legends focusing on the values inherent in depictions of psychopathic killers, quietly "mad" neighbors, victims who go insane, and others. Taken as a group and read as parallel texts, these narratives construct and present a complex of images of mental health and illness set in changing historical and cultural contexts. Together, the narratives create explanatory categories for mental illness and demonstrate popular understandings of "madness"; they equate insanity with visibility of difference, they explore the gendered associations of male aggression and female passivity, and they pinpoint areas of socially tolerable and intolerable deviance.

Of course, by taking the narratives as a parallel complex, the subtleties of culturally situated meanings may be sacrificed for the sake of constructing what appear to be universal patterns. This is always problematic, but all the more so in the exploration of concepts of deviance and abnormality, categories that are culturally defined on the basis of those behaviors understood as significantly and meaningfully divergent within a given social group. Clearly, what is treated as mental illness in one society could be considered criminal in another, or sinful in another, and as Nancy Scheper Hughes noted some time ago, that very same behavior might elsewhere "be understood as a mark of holy or privileged status" (1979:79). For this reason, the method used here is likely to only pick up on big pictures, lacking in the subtleties of cultural interpretation. It is worth noting, however, that images of mental illness in legend, as in film, TV, and literature, are largely about the big picture[5]—about creating differences that are large enough and visible enough to make us (the wishful and hopeful sane) feel, in contrast, safely and smugly normal. Visibility is crucial in these narratives. And, in fact, above all else, this is an essay about visibility and invisibility.

The Visible: Psychopathic Killers

There is good evidence that society (much like folklorists) reads legend, fiction, and those narratives provided by the popular media as parallel texts or as overlapping accounts leading to a larger and symbolically meaningful picture. Media analysts indicate that one in every eleven TV shows depicts a person labeled mentally ill, that 70 percent of those characters are characterized as violent, and that one-fifth are portrayed as killers (see Wahl 1995). One American study of the content included in top crime news copy found that the most likely elements were (1) insanity (especially psychopathic killers and homicidal maniacs); (2) unpredictability (especially multiple personalities and mild-mannered loners who commit criminal acts); and (3) the victimization of ordinary, unsuspecting people. The study concluded that "nothing sells newspapers like an insane, unpredictable, sudden gory killer on the loose" (Wahl 1995:111). The same might be said for what sells legend.[6]

The Hook,[7] the Choking Doberman,[8] and the Hairy-Handed Hitchhiker[9] are all examples of portrayals of psychopathic killers in legend, but all share another significant feature. In each of these stories, some physical characteristic becomes the visible sign of implied mental illness. Take, for example, the following narrative, from the Folklore Archives at the University of California, Berkeley, cited in Bill Ellis's article, "'The Hook' Reconsidered: Problems in Classifying and Interpreting Adolescent Horror Legends":

> Well, it seems this guy had lost his arm in an accident or something, so all
> he had was this big metal hook. And after, it happened his girlfriend ditched
> him.... Anyhow, he went crazy and started to take it out on everybody because
> he was jealous and he used to come up here where couples would be neck-
> ing. And he'd sneak up and open the door and hook the guy to death and then
> rape the girl.... Well, one night this couple was necking and the girl got really
> nervous and wanted to leave. Her boyfriend didn't want to but she wouldn't
> let him touch her or anything she was so upset. So he got really pissed and just

slammed the car in gear and revved out. And when he got to her house he went around to let her out and there was this hook hanging from the door.[10] (1994:61)

Legends such as the Hook superimpose images of physical disability over mental disability. The hook becomes the immediate sign that one is dealing with a psychopath. Other narratives resort to the same convention. In the collections at the Utah State University archives is a legend about a man with needle teeth. The story indicates that a woman meets a man in a bar and begins talking to him. After a while he smiles at her and she sees that his teeth are all made of needles. Frightened for her safety, she flees the bar and flags down a taxi on the street. After getting in the car she pours her heart out to the driver, telling him how frightened she was and all about the man with needle teeth she had left behind in the bar. The driver was unable to get a word in until her whole story was told. Meanwhile, they are far from busy streets, and when the driver eventually turns, he smiles and bears his own full mouth of needles.[11] While it is never said that the Needle Man is a psychopath, the story clearly indicates through her fear and through the described arrival of the car on less populated streets that we are meant to understand the driver to be demented and violent.

The Hook and the Needle Man share in common the notion that mental illness is coded on the physical body. Such a notion draws distinctions between the mentally healthy and the mentally ill in a direct and powerful way, creating easily identifiable ways of demarcating difference. Legend here falls within the same tradition as artistic renderings of male insanity, which traditionally emphasized the insane male as ugly, ferocious, bent over, cross-eyed, and bestial (Cross 2004; Gilman 1982). The notion that individuals who are identified as socially deviant are physically different than those seen as normal is a strangely recurring idea that has taken on many forms in Western scientific and popular thought. Certainly, the eighteenth-century focus on physiognomy, developed by Swiss preacher Johann Lavater, focused on the individual's inherent physical characteristics—the shape of a nose, the color of the eyes, or shape of the head—as characteristics which predetermined morality and the predisposition to mental illness (Gilman 1982; Lavater 1860). By the end of the eighteenth century, it was a commonplace belief that forms of insanity could be identified by the physical appearance of the afflicted. Medical historian Roy Porter notes,

> Ever since Antiquity, the theories of physiognomy, humours and complexions developed by Greek medicine fed the assumption that madness was as madness looked. Melancholics would be passive, listless, withdrawn, broadcasting the

black looks produced by black bile or the melancholic humour. Maniacs would resemble the brutes to whose bestial condition their inordinate voices had reduced them." (1991:92)

By the nineteenth century, the belief that moral character and mental stability were reflected in physical features led to efforts to measure the ears of criminals and the facial contours of those marked as deviants. With incredible tenaciousness, similar ideas have held on into the present. Sander Gilman, author of a number of volumes on the depiction of insanity in art and literature, argues, in reference to illness in general,

> Disease with its seeming randomness is one aspect of the indeterminable universe that we wish to distance from ourselves. To do so we must construct boundaries between ourselves and those categories of individuals whom we believe (or hope) to be more at risk than ourselves. Thus in contemporary . . . (culture) there is an assumption [even] among physicians, that the diseased and the beautiful cannot be encapsulated in one and the same category. (1988:1)

A friend who works as a psychiatric nurse indicated to me, in the same vein, that it is commonplace in psychiatric literature and in mental health worker vernacular tradition to assume that a trained professional will be able to see mental disorder in the eyes or facial expressions of their patients. Gilman continues,

> The tradition of visually representing madness in the form of various icons . . . whether body type, gesture or dress, point toward the need of society to identify the mad absolutely. . . . Thus the strength of the visual stereotype is in its immediacy. One does not even have to wait for the insane to speak. The mad are instantly recognizable, and it is our need for instantaneous awareness . . . which is the rationale for the visual stereotype. (48)

The ugly, disabled, and monster-like psychopath thus transcends the legend/ reality and media divide. Elaborating on an assertion made by the prosecution during the trial of serial killer Ted Bundy that "criminals are human beings and not hunchbacked cross-eyed monsters leaving a trail of slime," Stephen Michaud and Hugh Aynesworth, Bundy's biographers wrote:

> But with Ted Bundy, human being, that slithering hunchback lives, residing behind what one eminent psychiatrist has termed a psychopath's mask of sanity. The mask is a fabrication and nothing more, but it is impenetrable by even

the most skilled doctor of the mind. In Ted, the cross-eyed creature lurks on a different plane of existence and can only be seen by means of a tautology; its presence must be inferred before it can be found. . . . Only by means of his astounding capacity to compartmentalize had Bundy been able to keep the hunchback from raging through the mask and destroying him. When at last it did, Ted became the hunchback. No longer its protector, he and the entity fused. (Michaud and Aynesworth 1989:6, 13)

While the Hook, the Needle Man, and the Ted Bundy trial share in common the portrayal of the psychopathic killer as physically identifiable and monstrous, other legends more subtly code the physical body with criminality and insanity. Legends such as the Choking Doberman, while commonly focused on a slightly less monstrous criminal intent on burglary rather than murder, nevertheless leave the criminal body marked, missing the several fingers found in the throat of the choking dog. Although the message of the story addresses vulnerability of the lone individual comfortable in the safety of dog protection, the secondary message brands the criminal, forcing him to wear on his body physical signs of mental instability. Taken a step further and perhaps pushing the envelope a bit too far, one wonders about the marking of the castrated boy or the victim of kidney theft,[12] both suffering permanent body brands in exchange for the breaking of a social taboo—the child sent too young to use public facilities alone in the castrated boy legend, and the man too trusting of a stranger met in a bar in the kidney theft narrative.

Invisible Women

In general, though, these portrayals of mental illness in legend are gendered. Men are depicted in large terms as psychopathic killers and as deviant minds coded on deviant bodies. They are the big picture I referred to earlier, the highly visible, monstrously observable insane—who wear, in some sense, the mark of the devil. In contrast, mentally ill women, like the woman who reads the Welcome to the World of AIDS note or who eats the fried rat, go quietly, traumatically, and completely insane. They are victims not villains, and they are passive, not active. They are not made visible, but rather, they become invisible. Like the women in the AIDS story and the rat story, crazy women are carted away, banished to insane asylums. But they are also made invisible in other ways—hidden in their homes or sometimes turned into ghosts.[13] With women, we see them go crazy, but once they are crazy they are removed from the picture. Correspondingly, the catalyst for men to go crazy is rarely depicted, but their insane activities become the subject of the legendary events. In other words, according to the stories, women become crazy and disappear, men just are crazy and as a result become supervisible.

Surveying hundreds of contemporary legends, I was unable to locate even one monstrous female psychopathic killer, either in standard or in local legend. La Llorona, the weeping woman legend from Hispanic tradition, depicts a woman who goes crazy and kills her children (or kills her children and then goes crazy), but the representation is quite different than the hypervisible male killer. Bacil Kirtley cites the following version from Costa Rica:[14]

> In the dead of night, the country folk say, a sad voice calls for the attention of passersby. A beautiful country girl, it is said, was taken into service, brought to the capital, and there seduced by a young reprobate of the aristocracy. The girl returned home to have her baby. She drowned the infant in a creek and soon afterward went mad. Her cry is heard at night as she searches the creek and branches for her lost child. (Kirtley 1960:157)

And Pamela Jones collected the following collaborative version from two sisters-in-law in Oregon:

> ROSALBA: There was a woman who always went out at night and left all of her children at home alone. She would go out dancing and leave the children. She loved to go dancing. She was a *mujer libre*, a woman of the streets. Well one night she came home and her children were all gone and she was weeping and weeping and looking all over for them. She finally found her children, all dead, thrown over a cliff into an arroyo. And that is how you can hear the woman crying up and down the arroyo, looking for her children.
>
> ANTONIA: No, no, no, didn't *she* kill her children?
>
> ROSALBA: No, someone else came, and took them away.
>
> ANTONIA: Oh no. I am sure that *she* threw her children into the arroyo and then she went crazy (she twirls her finger by her ear) and spent all of her time wandering up and down the arroyos weeping and weeping and sometimes you can still hear her weeping in the arroyos. (Jones 1988:199)

But La Llorona is rarely described as monstrous. To the contrary, the legend casts a sympathetic eye on the murders—most often described as a response to the actions of an unfaithful lover, as a result of poverty, from an inability to look after her children or protect them from an abusive father. She is a victim in most versions, and although in the tradition she hunts down other people's children to replace her own, she is remorseful and grieving. She is, after all, the weeping woman.

Women who kill in legend generally kill children—like La Llorona or the teenage babysitter who roasts the baby.[15] But there is always a mediating factor—in the former case often the desire to protect the children, in the latter drugs or alcohol. But La Llorona *is* depicted as crazy. The narratives note her sudden and traumatic loss of sanity. From Shirley Arora's collections for example, one narrative noted that: "when her lover rejected her, she went out of her mind and drowned his children in the river. After her death she was compelled to search for them every night. Nowadays she appears like a ghost near watery places and on the streets, screaming and crying, 'Oh my children.'" Another notes that "she is a widow whose only son was lost playing near a flooded river. Insane from grief, she seeks to kidnap any small child she sees" (Arora 1981:25). La Llorona's grief-inspired insanity is consistent with the passive and melancholic image of women's madness, which like its monstrous male counterpart, appears to recur in cultural expression. Traced in its earliest manifestations to medieval art and literature, notions of melancholia understood as "love sickness" (Gilman 1982; Schiesari 1992) resulted in depictions of women's madness as quiet, passive, and despondent. Men, on the other hand, were depicted as highly agitated and dangerous in their insanity, exhibiting the three most agitated states of mind associated in the Middle Ages with mental illness—mania, epilepsy, and frenzy (Gilman 1982). Although La Llorona kills her children and steals those of others, there is a passiveness and victim-like nature to her activities. She is beside herself with mourning and, in many versions, does not choose by herself to steal but rather is condemned to wander the earth looking for her children.

It is difficult to find other examples to support observations concerning the active or passive nature of female insanity in legend because, as noted earlier, legendary women go crazy and then go away. These women are certainly not active, as their male counterparts are, but perhaps they have reached the height of passivity by simply fading away. Women like the lady who eats the rat in the Kentucky Fried Rat legend and the one who reads the note in Welcome to the World of AIDS are removed from narrative events and carted off to insane asylums. La Llorona kills herself in her insanity and can only come back as a ghost. The potentially murderous AIDS Mary (as some legend scholars have called the woman who leaves the "Welcome" message) leaves her message on the mirror and disappears (Goldstein 2004). Even in local legend, the crazy cat lady or community witch is rarely seen, being hidden behind doors and curtains. In contrast to the screaming visibility of male insanity, female insanity is invisible—removed from the community gaze. Like Brontë's madwoman in the attic in *Jane Eyre* or Charlotte Gilman's *The Yellow Wallpaper*,[16] the legendary madwoman is hidden from our view.

Moving from Invisible to Visible and Visible to Invisible: Hidden Madmen

But what of hiding madmen? Madmen certainly do hide in legend—the Hairy-Armed Hitchhiker, the Stranger Upstairs,[17] the Rapist Batman in the Closet,[18] the man under the bed in the Humans Can Lick Too story,[19] and numerous others, keep the madmen from our eyes.[20] However, in many of these stories, in contrast to the women's narratives, the man hides first and then is seen, whereas women are seen first and then disappear. Men go from invisible to visible, women do the reverse. But there is more there to intrigue us.

Let's look at the Hairy-Handed Hitchhiker. A lone woman driver gives a lift to an elderly woman. When the driver looks more closely at the woman she notes to her horror that the passenger's hands and arms are extraordinarily hairy. Realizing that she must have a man disguised as a woman in the car, the driver creates a pretense to ask the hitchhiker to get out (to check tires or to get a map). The driver speeds off once the passenger is out of the car. Later the police find the hitchhiker's handbag in the backseat and it contains a hatchet or meat cleaver.

Here we have another murderous madman—but in this case he is hiding, and significantly, he is dressed like a woman. The Hairy-Handed Hitchhiker and other hiding or invisible madmen are almost always feminized: they wear dresses (or tights in the Batman story), and they inhabit domestic spaces (or spaces more domesticated than are typical for legend locations), like the stranger upstairs or the criminal under the bed in the Humans Can Lick Too stories. As Steve Winick argues, concerning the Batman story, "it is probably not coincidental that Batman's hiding place is a closet and that to pose a threat to society he 'comes out of the closet'" (1992:21).

Passive-seeming, hiding, disturbed loner-type serial killers are also feminized in popular culture, academic literature, and the media. The fictional serial killer is often portrayed as suffering from gender confusion, usually attributed to neglectful or abusive mothering, and projects a feminine affect, sometimes exhibiting a tendency to cross dress (exemplified by Norman Bates in Alfred Hitchcock's *Psycho* as well as Jame Gumb in *Silence of the Lambs*), attacks in monthly lunar menstrual-type cycles, or wears the breasts or hair of his female victims (Grixti 1995:91). Gordene MacKenzie notes that the cross-dressing killer in popular culture exemplifies an extraordinary reversal, since statistically the cross-dressed man is far more likely to be slain by a psycho killer than to be one. The stereotype of the feminized cross-dressing mad killer, while it keeps the insanity hidden from the community gaze, simultaneously comments on gender and sexual orientation and marks the mentally ill person. Again, it responds to our need to have the insane be identifiable. As Gilman (1988:13) and others note, the real surprise is when the killer or mad bomber is the "guy next door" or the sweet meek man whom you see going to work each day. The mundane, quotidian killer is inconsistent with our need to have the mad person be identifiable, and therefore different from us. The surprise is when they are not different and not distinguishable.

The hidden insane woman is not the same as the hidden insane male. She is removed from our gaze not transformed with it—institutionalized, ghostly, hidden behind curtains and in attics. While we want desperately to see the mentally ill male, make him identifiable, we want equally desperately for female insanity to vanish.

Mental Illness, Visibility, and Gendered Truths

To some extent, these images are grounded in reality. Mental health statistics indicate that twice as many women as men suffer from depression, anxiety disorders, and eating disorders—all relatively passive illnesses (Usher 1991). But more men than women suffer from schizophrenia (Aleman, Kahn, and Selten 2003)—a far more active and potentially violent illness when left untreated (see Walsh, Buchanan, and Fahy 2002). Likewise, there is good reason to believe that mentally ill women have been somewhat invisible.

Following World War II, the United States, Canada, Britain, Australia, and other countries began to reform their psychiatric care systems based on new ideas of the adequate and humane treatment of mental illness. The recognition that isolation and confinement was not the answer for the treatment of all mental illnesses, combined with the development in the 1950s of antipsychotic drugs, led to the deinstitutionalization movement. Over the next four decades, hundreds of thousands of patients were released from government-run mental hospitals. Many of these patients returned to their families or were transferred to equally questionable conditions in nursing homes or boarding homes, but large numbers of individuals had no place to go and no real means of employment and, as a result, ended up on the streets. The deinstitutionalization movement, while initiated with the best of intentions, created a massive homeless problem, making huge numbers of mentally ill individuals previously locked away in hospitals suddenly a part of the community. The rise in stories of psychopathic killers and mentally ill villains in the media and popular culture has been traced by media scholars to the deinstitutionalization effort, which created a new kind of visibility for mental illness (see Cross 2014).

That visibility, however, was not gender neutral. Skid rows of the 1950s and 1960s were largely male enclaves, places where homeless men could jointly scrounge for shelter, food, and odd bits of employment. The maleness of skid rows skewed the literature on homelessness, defining it as a male problem and demonstrating only recognition of male homeless circumstances and strategies for survival. Feminist research and literature on homelessness produced over the past twenty years stresses that there have always been homeless women, but that unlike their male counterparts, their significant numbers have been hidden from the public view. The political scientist Paul Higate (2000) suggests that "attempts to understand . . . homelessness . . . might [usefully] be considered from the perspective of gender" and concludes that "in a heuristic sense, this could [best] be represented by men occupying a highly visible 'rough sleeping' position . . . [and] women . . . [as being] amongst the 'hidden homeless' population" (332).

Similarly, Sophie Watson and Helen Austerberry state, "there is a strong case for the argument that an unquantifiable proportion of women's potential homelessness remains concealed" (1986:83). Sociologist Michael Martin makes the same observation. He writes, "Although homeless women . . . have existed since the beginning of recorded history, they have been politely 'not seen.'. . . Consequently very little is known about their experiences" (1987:33). Claudia Hirst, explaining a statistic that identified twice as many homeless males as females during the late 1980s in Melbourne, argues that men are more visibly homeless and that more young women fall into the category of the hidden homeless than do men (Hirst 1989). Fearing vulnerability to street violence, particularly sexual violence, and often accompanied by children, women without homes do not cluster in the same way as men, but rather find ways to hide away, preferring the safety of concealment rather than the power of numbers (Harter 2005; May and Johnson 2007; Watson 1999). The North American association with women that we do see living on the streets is the "bag lady," a woman who carries all of her worldly belongings around with her in bags or in a shopping cart. Men who do the same are still regarded as "homeless men," while the bag lady title remains the nomenclature for females, objectifying their homelessness. While homeless men are taken to be potentially violent, homeless women are often characterized as eccentric but harmless. Our desire to think of them as not truly homeless, as invisible from the streets at least at night, or in the potential future, is captured in the numerous legends concerning great stashes of money that they might have hidden away in their bags,[21] in bus lockers, or even in mansions.

But grounded in reality or not, the notion of the supervisible mentally ill male versus the invisible mentally ill woman still begs the question of "Why?" Certainly, from a feminist perspective, women remain invisible in many areas requiring social services, falling through the cracks of male-dominated definitions of social problems. But if we return to the narrative effort to mark the mentally ill as different from us, one wonders if women, by virtue of their role in birth and nurturing, become in some sense representative of reproduction, representative, in other words, of all of us. To make the mentally ill woman visible perhaps calls into question our own stability. If we make her monstrous, do we call into place questions about our own potential monstrosity?

What is clear is that we fear the crossing of the delicate sanity/insanity divide. Several other legends make this concern apparent. In one, a famous chef named Napoleon is loaned to a friend to cook a special dinner. He carefully wraps his gourmet cooking knives in newspaper to carry with him. When his car breaks down en route to the friend's house, he quickly runs to catch a bus. In his haste, the chef jostles his bundle of knives enough so that as he boards, the bus driver catches sight of a meat cleaver. The bus driver, fearing for his own safety, drives the chef to the local mental hospital. Thinking this must be his intended destination, the chef unwraps his knives and announces, "I'm Napoleon, where's the party?"[22]

In a second story, a bus driver carrying twenty mental patients from an outing back to their hospital decides to stop to have a drink. When he returns to his bus, he discovers that all of the patients have escaped. Desperate for a solution, the driver stops at the next public bus stop and offers a free ride to all those waiting. He then delivers his new passengers to the mental hospital, where they are promptly given medication and returned to their rooms.[23] Other related legends portray psychology students given an assignment to mimic symptoms and fake their way into psychiatric care. Of course, they succeed so well that they are institutionalized. By the time their instructor comes to explain, the students, who are now heavily sedated, have themselves descended into madness (Rosenhan 1974).

The concern with the sane being easily mistaken for the insane clearly articulates our desire to draw clear boundaries between the healthy observer and patient. The stories, however, betray with equal clarity the very scary notion that this boundary is fragile and that, like the lady in the AIDS story or like the woman who eats the rat, we might suddenly and completely find ourselves on the other side. In this sense, while the narratives are heavily stereotyped and often cruel, they are simultaneously acutely aware of the thin line between them and us, a line that delineates the right to visibility or invisibility.

Notes

1. Welcome to the World of AIDS appears in other variants. For more information on the narrative, see Goldstein (2004).

2. These narratives were collected when HIV was generally understood as terminal and not yet a chronic manageable disease.

3. The Boyfriend's Death refers to a legend in which a young couple runs out of gas. The boyfriend leaves with a gas can and goes looking for a gas station. The girlfriend hears on the radio that there is a violent patient who has escaped from a nearby asylum. Frightened, she locks all doors. After a while, she hears scratching on the car windows. She turns the radio up louder and tries to ignore the sound, but eventually gets out to remove a tree branch she thinks is scratching the car. When she gets out, she sees the gas can lying on the ground and her boyfriend hanging from the tree with his fingernails worn down and bloody. See Brunvand (1999:103–4).

4. A mother allows her little boy to go alone into a men's public washroom for the first time instead of going with her into the ladies'. When he does not return, she asks a man nearby to go in and look for him. He finds the little boy in a pool of blood with his penis cut off. See Brunvand (1984:82–92).

5. See Wilson (1998:89–95) for the interface between legend and the press.

6. Numerous studies have demonstrated that patients discharged from psychiatric facilities who did not abuse alcohol and illegal drugs had a rate of violence no different than that of their neighbors in the community but were far more likely to become victims of violence than were others in the general population. See Corrigan, Rowan et al. (2002).

7. The Hook legend generally takes the form of a lover's lane narrative about a couple who, while making out in the car, hear a bulletin on the radio about an escaped violent inmate from the local asylum. He is described as having a hook for a prosthesis. The couple hears noises from the car door and quickly activate the locks. They peel out of the spot where they are parked. Arriving home, they find a bloody hook hanging from the door handle. See Brunvand (2001a:200–1).

8. Once again, a news report indicates that a violent killer has escaped from the local prison asylum. A woman leaves her house to go to the theater and forgets to lock her door. Coming home, she finds her dog choking in the hallway. She rushes to the vet, who performs tracheal surgery only to find three human fingers in the dog's throat. She leaves the vet and goes home to discover a trail of blood leading to her bedroom closet. In her closet is the escaped inmate, missing fingers and passed out from blood loss. See Brunvand (1984:3–18).

9. The Hairy-Handed Hitchhiker, also referred to as the Hairy-Armed Hitchhiker, is a story about a woman who picks up a female hitchhiker but notices out of the corner of her

eye that the "woman" has exceedingly large and hairy hands and arms. She stops at a gas station and asks the woman to go in and get her a Coke. As soon as "she" leaves the car, the driver locks the door and speeds off to the local police station. In her car the police find the hitchhiker's purse, which contains a bloody ax. See Brunvand (1986:157–59).

10. Interviewer comments, marked by ellipses, have been removed from this reproduction of the text. For the original with comments, see Ellis (1994).

11. From the Fife Folklore Archives, Utah State University, Logan, Utah.

12. The Kidney Theft is a narrative about a traveling man or woman who goes to the hotel bar for a drink. He or she meets a stranger and they have a drink. The next thing the traveler knows, he or she is waking up in the hotel in a bathtub full of ice. Taped to the mirror is a note telling the traveler to call 911. The 911 operator tells the traveler that he or she is the latest in a rash of crimes for kidney harvesting. See Brunvand (1993:149–54).

13. Jeannie Banks Thomas notes that supernatural manifestations of deviant crazy women are a common pattern in ghost stories (Goldstein, Grider, and Thomas 2008:81–110).

14. Originally published in Victor H. Lizano, *Leyendas de Costa Rica* (San Jose, Costa Rica, 1941), 105–107.

15. A stoned babysitter puts the baby in the oven and the turkey in the crib. See Brunvand (2001b:55).

16. First published in 1892, "The Yellow Wallpaper" is a short story by Charlotte Stetson Perkins (Gilman) about a woman who is confined by her husband to an upstairs room to recuperate from depression. The confinement, without stimulation, creates a kind of psychosis in which she becomes obsessed with both the wallpaper and the color yellow.

17. The Stranger Upstairs is the story of a babysitter who gets a series of phone calls from a man asking if she has checked the children. She calls the police, who trace the stranger's calls. They immediately call back and tell her to get the kids out of the house immediately because the calls are coming from inside the house. They are too late and the kids have already been brutally murdered. See Brunvand (1981:54–57).

18. A man goes home with a woman; she ties him to the bed as a prelude for sex but then leaves the room. A man dressed as Batman busts out of the closet and rapes the man. See Winick (1992:1–21).

19. A young girl is home alone and hears on the radio that a violent killer has escaped from the asylum. She goes to bed with her trusty dog on the floor near her. Several times during the night she awakes to a dripping sound. Too scared to get up, she reaches down and feels her dog lick her hand. Reassured, she falls back asleep. The next morning she still hears the dripping coming from the bathroom. She goes in and finds her dog with his throat cut in the shower. On the mirror written in blood is a note saying "humans can lick too." See Brunvand (2001a:241).

20. The costume motif that appears in the Batman story is common. The story of Bunny Man, popular in Washington DC, Virginia, and Maryland describes a crazed killer dressed in a bunny costume who attacks people with an ax (see Blank and Puglia 2014:58–60). In some versions of the narrative, the transfer of patients from an asylum ends in a crashed bus. Bunny Man escapes from the vehicle only to terrorize nearby residents and travelers. Thank you to Trevor Blank for reminding me of this example.

21. This story about some well-known homeless woman has existed in every city in which I have lived.

22. Reported in http://www.snopes.com/medical/asylum/crazybus.asp (accessed September 2009).

23. Ibid. See also Rosenhan (1974).

References

Aleman André, René S. Kahn, and Jean-Paul Selten. 2003. "Sex Differences in the Risk of Schizophrenia: Evidence from Meta-analysis." *Archives General of Psychiatry* 60 (6):565–81.

Arora, Shirley L. 1981. "La Llorona: The Naturalization of a Legend." *Southwest Folklore* 5 (1):23–40.

Aynesworth, Hugh, Ted Bundy, and Michaud Stephen. 2000. *Ted Bundy: Conversations with a Killer.* Irving, TX: Authorlink Press.

Blank, Trevor J., and David J. Puglia. 2014. *Maryland Legends: Folklore from the Old Line State.* Charleston, SC: The History Press.

Brunvand, Jan Harold. 1984. *The Choking Doberman.* New York: W. W. Norton.

———. 1986. *The Mexican Pet.* New York: W. W. Norton.

———. 1993. *The Baby Train.* New York: W. W. Norton.

———. 1999. *Too Good to Be True: The Colossal Book of Urban Legends.* New York: W. W. Norton.

———. 2001a. *Encyclopedia of Urban Legends* New York: W. W. Norton.

———. 2001b. *The Truth Never Stands in the Way of a Good Story.* Urbana: University of Illinois Press.

Caputi, Jane. 1993. "American Psychos: The Serial Killer in Contemporary Fiction." *Journal of American Culture* 16 (4):101–12.

Corrigan, Patrick W., David Rowan, Amy Green, Robert Lundin, Philip River, Kyle Uphoff-Wasowski, Kurt White, and Mary Anne Kubiak. 2002. "Challenging Two Mental Illness Stigmas: Personal Responsibility and Dangerousness." *Schizophrenia Bulletin* 28 (2):293–309.

Cross, Simon. 2004. "Visualizing Madness: Mental Illness and Public Representation." *Television & New Media* 5 (3):197–216.

———. 2014. "Mad and Bad Media: Populism and Pathology in the British Tabloids." *European Journal of Communication* 20 (10):1–14.

Ellis, Bill. 1994. "'The Hook' Reconsidered: Problems in Classifying and Interpreting Adolescent Horror Legends." *Folklore* 105:61–75.

Fine, Gary Alan. 1992. *Manufacturing Tales: Sex and Money in Contemporary Legends.* Knoxville: University of Tennessee Press.

Gilman, Sander L. 1982. *Seeing the Insane.* Lincoln: University of Nebraska Press.

———. 1988. *Disease and Representation: Images of Illness from Madness to AIDS.* Ithaca, NY: Cornell University Press.

Goldstein, Diane E. 2004. *Once Upon a Virus: AIDS Legends and Vernacular Risk Perception*. Logan: Utah State University Press.

Goldstein, Diane E., Sylvia Ann Grider, and Jeannie Banks Thomas. 2008. *Haunting Experiences: Ghosts in Contemporary Folklore*. Logan: Utah State University Press.

Goss, Michael. 1990. "The Halifax Slasher and Other 'Urban Maniac' Tales." In *A Nest of Vipers: Perspectives on Contemporary Legend*, vol. 5, ed. Gillian Bennett and Paul Smith, 89–112. Sheffield, UK: University of Sheffield Academic Press.

Grixti, Joseph. 1995. "Consuming Cannibals: Psychopathic Killers as Archetypes and Cultural Icons." *Journal of American Culture* 18 (1):87–96.

Harper, Stephen. 2005. "Media, Madness and Misrepresentation: Critical Reflections on Anti-Stigma Discourse." *European Journal of Communication* 20 (4):460–83.

Harter, Lynn M., Charlene Berquist, B. Scott Titsworth, David Novak, and Tod Brokaw. 2005. "The Structuring of Invisibility among the Hidden Homeless: The Politics of Space, Stigma, and Identity Construction." *Journal of Applied Communication Research* 33 (4):305–27.

Hartley, Lucy. 2001. *Physiognomy and the Meaning of Expression in Nineteenth-Century Culture*. Cambridge: Cambridge University Press.

Higate, Paul. 2000. "Ex-servicemen on the Road: Travel and Homelessness." *Sociological Review* 48 (3):331–47.

Hirst, Claudia, David Stephens, and Anne Houlihan. 1989. *Forced Exit: A Profile of the Young Homeless in Inner Urban Melbourne*. Melbourne, Australia: Salvation Army Youth Homelessness Policy Development Project.

Jones, Pamela. 1988. "'There Was a Woman': La Llorona in Oregon." *Western Folklore* 47 (3):195–211.

Kirtley, Bacil F. 1960. "'La Llorona' and Related Themes." *Western Folklore* 19 (3):155–68.

Lavater, Johann Caspar. 1860. *Essays on Physiognomy*. London: R. Worthington.

MacKenzie, Gordene Olga. 1994. *Transgender Nation*. Bowling Green, OH: Bowling Green State University Popular Press.

Martin, Michael. 1987. "Homeless Women: An Historical Perspective." In *On Being Homeless: Historical Perspectives*, ed. Rick Beard, 32–41. New York: Museum of the City of New York.

May, Jon, Paul Cloke, and Sarah Johnsen. 2007. "Alternative Cartographies of Homelessness: Rendering Visible British Women's Experiences of 'Visible' Homelessness." *Gender, Place and Culture* 14 (2):121–40.

Porter, Roy, ed. 2003. *The Faber Book of Madness*. London: Faber & Faber.

Rosenhan, David L. 1974. "On Being Sane in Insane Places." *Clinical Social Work Journal* 2 (4):237–56.

Scheper-Hughes, Nancy. 2001. *Saints, Scholars, and Schizophrenics: Mental Illness in Rural Ireland*. Berkeley: University of California Press.

Schiesari, Juliana. 1992. *The Gendering of Melancholia: Feminism, Psychoanalysis, and the Symbolics of Loss in Renaissance Literature*. Ithaca, NY: Cornell University Press.

Stetson (Gilman), Charlotte Perkins. 1892. "The Yellow Wall-paper. A Story." *The New England Magazine* 11 (5):647–57.

Usher, Jane M. 1991. *Women's Madness: Misogyny or Mental Illness?* Amherst: University of Massachusetts Press.

Wahl, Otto F. 1995. *Media Madness: Public Images of Mental Illness.* New Brunswick, NJ: Rutgers University Press.

Walsh, Elizabeth, Alec Buchanan, and Thomas Fahy. 2002. "Violence and Schizophrenia: Examining the Evidence." *British Journal of Psychiatry* 180 (6):490–95.

Watson, Sophie, and Helen Austerberry. 1986. *Housing and Homelessness: A Feminist Perspective.* London: Routledge and Kegan Paul.

Watson, Susan. 1999. "Home Is Where the Heart Is: Engendering Notions of Homelessness." In *Homelessness: Exploring the New Terrain*, ed. Patricia Kennett and Alex Marsh, 81–100. Bristol, UK: Policy Press.

Wilson, Michael. 1998. "Legend and Life: 'The Boyfriend's Death' and 'The Mad Axeman.'" *Folklore* 109 (1–2):89–95.

Winick, Stephen. 1992. "Batman in the Closet: A New York Legend." *Contemporary Legend* 2:1–21.

CHAPTER EIGHT

Broadcasting the Stigmatized Self: Positioning Functions of YouTube Vlogs on Bipolar Disorder[1]

—Darcy Holtgrave

Once or twice a week, a young woman who goes by the name Desa Kroma turns a video camera on herself.[2] Most often she films from her bedroom, and behind her we see her nightstand with books, a brass lamp, and a few medication bottles. From this intimate space, Desa Kroma shares her thoughts and stories about her life. Starting in November 2013, she has made appearances on YouTube, the free Internet video sharing platform where her videos are publicly available. She has revealed many personal things: she is an artist, a cat owner, and a fan of the card game *Magic: The Gathering*, which inspired her username. The main thing she talks about, though, is her experience with bipolar disorder. She and I have never met face-to-face; rather, she has chosen freely to share a part of her life with me (and anyone else with access and interest) in the hopes that her videos have a beneficial effect, either for her or for her audience. And she is by no means alone.

I began exploring the ways that people talk about their personal experience with mental illness on the Internet as a matter of convenience. With a few clicks, I found blogs, discussion boards, and other forms of text-only communication that introduced me to some of the themes and ideas people talked about. I honed in on the topic of bipolar disorder, a mental illness characterized by abnormal shifts in mood,[3] in part because I had been prescribed a medication used to treat mood disorders (though bipolar disorder was not my diagnosis), but also because bipolar disorder seemed to be an increasingly common diagnosis.[4]

In my Internet wanderings, I came across YouTube. I quickly discovered that many people dedicate their endeavors to sharing stories about particular illnesses, including bipolar disorder. I currently follow over 180 people whose YouTube channels (pages where a viewer may access all of a person's publicly available videos) are dedicated entirely or largely to presenting their personal experience with bipolar disorder. Although more than half of my subscriptions—which were compiled from searches on the term *bipolar disorder* within YouTube as well as following others' subscriptions—consist of young white women from North America,[5] making videos on this topic is by no means solely an endeavor of that demographic; the people in my sample range in age from late teens to mid-sixties, and they come from a wide range of ethnicities and (mostly English-speaking) countries of origin.

In these videos, their creators sometimes reveal deeply personal things about themselves, both positive and negative—like the birth of a child or the thrill of finding love to abusive relationships or suicidal thoughts. They also sometimes talk about everyday things, like oil changes or grocery store trips, as if they were conversing with a friend. Some record their in-the-moment emotions, talking through a particular issue in a quasi-soliloquy that comes from addressing an imagined audience to a camera or the speaker's own image reflected in a computer monitor. Sometimes that in-the-moment emotion is boredom. "I can't think of what else to say," they sometimes declare, and then cast around until they do or turn the camera off.

While I did have contact with members of this community to inform them of my research, in my analysis here, I relied primarily on observations of publicly available speech and comments. My decision to remain an observer and not take a more active role in the community has not gone unexamined. A few considerations came into play. On YouTube, an observer is, in a sense, a participant, and these participants generally far outnumber the ones who actively comment or respond by another video (Buccitelli 2012:73–74). Video views influence the YouTube algorithm that decides whether a video is promoted or recommended in other viewers' feeds.[6] YouTube tracks and publishes how many times a video is viewed, and even minimal gestures like anonymously giving a video a "thumbs up" or a "thumbs down" show in a running tally below the video.[7] It goes without saying that behind-the-scenes communication between community members takes place.

For the sake of this introductory project, however, I discovered that there is rich and nuanced information—cogent and direct answers to questions I had formed—about experiences, opinions, and motivations for posting videos on YouTube that people already publicly volunteer in their videos and comments. The expressive genre that I am studying is founded on public introspection, and the video creators talk freely about all the topics that have appeared in this chapter. My goal here is to explore the ways individuals publicly use the platform of YouTube in the service of increasing awareness, providing information, and expressing themselves in order to benefit mental health. The genre in question, vlogging,[8] is an Internet folk film tradition that is characterized by people talking about their personal experience in a verbal diary-like form.[9]

An early version of YouTube's "About" page stated that the purpose of YouTube was to "Show off your favorite videos to the world/Take videos of your dogs, cats, and other pets/Blog the videos you take with your digital camera or cell phone/Securely and privately show videos to your friends and family around the world/ . . . and much, much more!" (Burgess and Green 2009:3). This lighthearted introduction does not suggest that something as weighty as a discussion of bipolar disorder could occur, but as Barbara Kirshenblatt-Gimblett observes:

> The specificity of networked interactive electronic communication becomes specially clear in the unintended consequences of non-instrumental uses of these media, uses for which they were not initially intended. For this reason, playful uses of the medium may be even more revealing than strictly practical applications, which are not without social and cultural consequences. (1996:22)

It seems Kirshenblatt-Gimblett's "playful use" of a "playful medium" becomes, in this case, a serious use of a medium: providing information and seeking and giving support on mental illness.

How computer-mediated communication is perceived by those who use it is the subject of a great deal of discussion by users and scholars alike. Trevor J. Blank notes how individuals "make connections with others in a simulative setting of tremendous intimacy" (2013:106–12). The perception of connection is just as immediate as an in-person context. That being given, the hybridized physical/virtual context (what Blank calls "virtual corporeality") allows for exposure and moves that are not possible in physical life.

What I see as a particular benefit of the vlogging form for the mental health community is how the asynchronous communication involved in responses (see Buccitelli 2012) provides the speaker with a locus of control that may be protective of sensitive, personal topics. YouTube performers receive audience reaction and feedback in a computer-mediated form, and they can choose to some extent the levels and kinds of interaction they have with audience members. Comments on videos can be set to appear automatically, without any review from the video owner; they can be subject to the video creator's approval; or they can be disabled, rendering it impossible for site patrons to comment whatsoever.[10] In addition, users may choose to make their email addresses or social media sites visible for further contact, or if users wish to post videos and receive no comments or emails, they may.

On the other hand, users lack control over the kinds of exposure they receive as a result of posting on YouTube. They post with the knowledge that YouTube is freely available (depending on the country) and most do not use or reveal their legal names; some even obscure their faces or post text- or voice-only videos in order to protect their privacy. While this may seem counter to the idea of openly talking about their disorder, the hazards associated with posting on the Internet are very real. For example, one vlogger, Bipolar Disorder Nerd, had his mental health advocacy videos shared on the channel where he used his real name:

> After I posted my last video, which kind of outlined the documentary that I'm trying to make about depression and suicide and mental illness, and I was asking for help getting it you know spread around, someone went on my public, you know, personal under my-own-name YouTube account and started posting this one, you know my, my bipolar vlog account which is full of all sorts of intimate stuff and started posting that one in comments and harassing me, posting all sorts of other weird, I don't know if they were attacks or insults, but totally random weird things, so I went back and made all 36 videos that were left on, on my blog channel private, and that's pretty much the end of this channel. And it's a good lesson, you know, don't put anything on the Internet you wouldn't what your mom, your boss, and your friends to see, so, yeah, but that's—I guess that's it. I mean no more, no more vlogging for me.[11]

In the interim, however, Bipolar Disorder Nerd had a change of heart and has since re-released many of his videos.

The core belief about the Internet as illustrated in the narratives of these vlogs is that the Internet—and, by extension, YouTube—is and should be a democratic venue for free expression. People believe that they have a right to express their beliefs and relate their experiences without censorship. Both passive viewing and active participation are valuable, but vloggers regularly encourage the audience members to actively participate in the form of subscriptions, comments, and private messages. YouTube's early tagline, "Broadcast Yourself," goes with the belief that getting the narrative out is beneficial to the speaker. "Broadcast Yourself" is a command, or an offer: "[This is a place where you can] Broadcast Your Self."

Vlogging as Positioning

Michael Bamberg's (1997) concept of narrative positioning applied to these narratives reveals the multilayered negotiations within vloggers' narratives. Positioning in conversation describes the interchanges in which speakers co-negotiate aspects of their identity (Bamberg 1997: 336). Although Bamberg works with synchronous, in-person interaction, the asynchronous conversation involved in the bipolar disorder vlogging communities—in which speakers actively tend comment fields across multiple videos, as well as preemptively in negotiations with an imagined audience—is filled with positioning moves in their "[concern] with self-reflection, self-criticism, and agency (all ultimately oriented toward the possibility of *self-revisions*)" (Bamberg 2005:224).

Bamberg proposes analyzing positioning from several vantage points; first, how characters within related events are placed in relation to each other, and then how speakers place themselves to the audience as well as to themselves (1997:336–37). Not all of the videos in my study necessarily report events; sometimes they summarize research or discuss emotional states. In videos wherein events are in fact reported, the vloggers describe interactions with others within their personal and professional life—partners, relatives, friends, instructors, coworkers. They also report on interactions with members of the medical community, including psychiatrists, psychologists, counselors, nurses, and admissions personnel. Finally, if we consider entities as characters, then vloggers also report interactions with organizations like insurance companies, billing agencies, and disability offices. Bamberg writes:

> This type of analysis aims at the linguistic means that do the job of marking one person as, for example, (a) the agent who is in control while the action is inflicted on another, or (b) as the central character who is helplessly at the mercy of outside (quasi "natural") forces, or who is rewarded by luck, fate, or personal qualities (such as bravery, nobility, or simply "character"). (1997:337)

The vloggers whose videos I have seen may present themselves as educators or examples. They may establish and head support networks. They may also position themselves as representatives, as public faces, who are willing to be vocal about their disorder and even work for rights. They may also position themselves as victims and sufferers, people who feel little agency against this disorder and the stigma it brings.

The Functions of Vlogging on Bipolar Disorder

Vlogging, like any expressive form, can serve particular functions, and of the 180+ vlog channels about bipolar disorder that I follow, four common functions are apparent: information sharing, community formation, promoting self-efficacy and healing, and mitigating stigma. These uses of this form of video communication come about in an underlying suggestion that narrative is a form of agency and a tool of healing for mental illness, combined with a complementary belief that the Internet in general, and YouTube in particular, is a context where freedom of speech should be allowed and encouraged. These vlogs are evidence of the belief that sharing one's personal story through narrative can have a positive impact on both the listener and the speaker.

Function 1: Providing Information

Most of the bipolar disorder vloggers in my sample provide a definition of bipolar disorder, and often within their first few videos. For the most part, these definitions are based on a Western biomedical model; vloggers directly quote from a variety of sources, from the medical field's *Diagnostic and Statistical Manual of Mental Disorders* (DSM-5)—which is used in medical diagnosing and billing—to popular sources like WebMD.com. The vlogger who goes by the name Rawsammi, for example, reads from a college textbook to define a mixed episode, which can occur in people with bipolar disorder:

> A mixed episode is characterized by symptoms of both a full-blown manic or major depressive episode for at least one week, whether the symptoms are intermixed or alternate rapidly every few days. . . . It's like depression on steroids . . . normally when you're depressed you're like, dulled out, but then when you're having a mixed episode, it's like, you can be in bed depressed but also your skin is crawling.[12]

Rawsammi suggests she is using the textbook definition for the sake of convenience and clarity; also, drawing upon authoritative sources positions her as well-informed and credible.[13] As personal experience confers authority on the topic of bipolar disorder, people sometimes put up their own experience as what to do or not do. Desa Kroma says, "You really have to fight against the current, that's the big thing I think I've learned from this whole recent experience . . . instead of running, you know, I think it's a better idea for me to try to calm down, watch a show, try to focus my energy, maybe try writing . . . and just try to relax."[14]

Users provide information about their experiences in certain circumstances—hospitalization, for example—in order to demystify it for viewers. Information about psychiatric medications, particularly in the form of user reviews, is also common. The two vloggers of Bipolardiscussions (a boyfriend-girlfriend team that creates videos as a couple and individually) have posted discussions of common prescription drugs administered for the treatment of bipolar and other mood disorders, such as Risperdal, Depakote, Seroquel, Zyprexa, and Zoloft. In one video, the woman says:

> I just wanted to do a quick review of some medications that I've taken for my bipolar [disorder] that really didn't help at all and made me feel like shit most of the time. Number one, and this will always be number one on my list, it'd have to be Risperdal, because I was a zombie on that stuff, and it did some weird, weird shit to my body.

This included dramatic weight gain, lactation, problems with her menstrual cycle, and lack of emotions.[15] The man talks about his own issues with it: "It gave me headaches, it made my internal organs hurt. . . . This is the nicest thing I can say about this medication, is it gave me an Adderall buzz for like ten seconds. What else? It made me suicidal and agitated, and I had to stop taking it on day three."[16] The man also gives medications colorful ratings, and Risperdal "gets one shredded tire that exploded on the freeway and caused a wreck, that's what it gets. . . . It gets one dead goldfish. And it gets a flaming pile of wires, that's my rating for Risperdal."[17]

The bipolar disorder vlogging community invokes several kinds of authority. Some quote from resources like the National Alliance for Mental Illness; others refer to Bible verses. The most crucial, central authority to the genre of bipolar disorder vlogs is of course the narrator him- or herself. Diane Goldstein's work with online support groups about menopause observes that in this kind of vernacular context, "the absence of medical authority allows for the creation of authority based on experience rather than based on 'objective' information" (2000:315). Voices from the medical community do appear on YouTube, but within the vloggers I am following, only two reveal they have any professional involvement with the medical field, and very few comments are offered from people saying they are healthcare professionals.

The main thing that supports that person's authority in this context is the personal experience narrative of mental illness. Ownership of that story is very clearly staked, and vloggers include in their videos verbal and textual reminders that it is their own experience with phrases like "my story," "my experience with," and "my personal experience with." These phrases remind the reader that the vlogger's experience is unique and also reinforce their authority.[18] Examples of titles include "Everything Bipolar: MY STORY. The beginning of my battle against bipolar disorder,"[19] "BIPOLAR DISORDER: My Story,"[20] and "My Bipolar Story."[21]

Statements asserting the vlogger's right to his or her opinion and point of view are also made. One vlogger uses her second video to respond to comments and questions on her first. In the introduction she states, "So, all of this is my personal opinion, again, please don't judge me based on my personal opinion because it will most likely differ from yours."[22] Another weighs in on medication: "I've been watching other people's videos on YouTube and whether they approve or disapprove of psych meds, and, I mean, everybody has their own opinion, I don't care either way if you choose to take them or not, it's absolutely none of my business. I personally choose to take them."[23]

The importance of the authority of personal experience becomes clearest when it is contested. Debates about models of illness rage on, but what is perhaps most cutting is not differing interpretations of the illness but, rather, a flat denial of that person's experience. For example, one comment that was left on a video said, "I don't believe you. You're bragging about a disorder and putting your 'diagnosis' on youtube. You're obviously attention starved and pretending to have an issue."[24] This kind of commentary is often met with outraged responses from the vlogger and other commentators defending the narrator's story and right to tell it.

In the economy where authenticity means authority, any doubt of the authenticity of a narrator's experience is detracting, particularly when the vlog is intended to help others. Rawsammi directly addresses this issue in her video, "Am I Credible?" She chooses three points—first, the veracity of the information she passes along; second, the truthfulness of the stories she reports; and third, the validity of the advice she dispenses:

> I do have a bachelors degree from a research university, prominent research university, called the University of Georgia. . . . And I finished two semesters of graduate school in public health and I feel like mental health issues is a public health issue, it's in the public domain of public health, so I feel like I can speak about this stuff. . . . And as far as my credibility for my personal experiences, you know, I guess that's just up for you to decide, and even if you do think it's an act, which it isn't, you know, you've got to give me credit for being creative, I guess, even though, honestly, I am not creative or smart enough to make that stuff up.[25]

Repeated telling of narratives and assurances from a vlogger that he or she is honest about the experiences with illness may do little to assuage a viewer's doubts, though. Western culture, namely its legal systems, values

documentation and testimonials as corroboration of the validity of a narrative (Bohmer and Shuman 2008:115–32). Vloggers key in to this when they
talk. Some show their hospital bracelets; others hold up their pill bottles.
SuperCrazylady21 creates a video that pans over release papers from her most
recent hospitalization, lingering on the medications and diagnosis:

> I'm tired of these trolls saying that I'm either possessed by some demon or that
> I'm a fake attention whore whatever. I am not a fake at all, and I have proof to
> show it [pans the camera over discharge papers]. . . . Now, here is some proof
> that I was inpatient. See that right there? . . . And it says "reason for hospitaliza-
> tion, mood stabilization and medication management," there's my shady fucking
> psychiatrist, and then there is my diagnoses. Which is schizoaffective disorder,
> attention deficit disorder, and post traumatic stress disorder. Oh my God! So
> apparently, you know, I'm a fake. I'm not a fucking fake.[26]

Function 2: Forming Community

Providing information and advice also serves as ways of forming community around the topic. Several state that they have started their channels in
attempts to begin support groups. SuperCrazylady21 writes in a comment on
one of her videos, "I make these videos for those who feel alone due to mental
diseases."[27] "You are not alone" is a reassuring statement frequently spoken in
the vlogging community on bipolar disorder. Implicit in this statement is the
assertion "*I* am not alone." Bipolar Disorder Nerd recognizes that the reason
he is making these videos in the first place is for community, and he ends one
video by stating, "If you like this, if you relate to any of this, drop a comment,
cause you know I could just make videos and keep them on my hard drive,
the reason I'm putting them on YouTube is because I want, I want to connect
with people, so if you feel some kind of connection with this, drop me a comment. Thanks."[28]

In thinking about the practice of watching and producing for YouTube,
which resembles watching and producing television, it may be difficult to
envision YouTube as a place of community interaction. Indeed, a channel
maintained by an individual user does not necessarily delineate a place of
community at the outset. The vlogger is the focal point of the video page;
he or she has the stage, and opportunity for interaction is relegated to the
comments fields or a tucked-away page of the channel's "Discussions" page.
Some critics even claim that celebrity-seeking is the site's primary function
(Kavoori 2011:17). In their book *YouTube: Online Video and Participatory*

Culture, Jean Burgess and Michael Green claim that YouTube's structures for personal interaction have not been as conducive to community-building in the ways that social media sites have become; however, they do argue that community-building within YouTube is possible, and the users that I have observed often state that they do feel a great sense of community. Users have simply had to be creative within the confines of the YouTube structure to create community through the open-ended abilities of search engines, tags, automated recommendations, and so on (Burgess and Green 2009:63–70). Rotman, Golbeck, and Preece note that "personal profile pages ('channels'), personal bulletin boards and comment sections, lists of friends, subscribers and favored users all enhance users' individual representation on the network, but do not bring large groups of users together"; rather, they "[form] an almost random network structure" (2009:47). I came to the bipolar disorder vlogs in my project from many different directions—searches, subscription trails, and so on—because, as Rotman, Golbeck, and Preece note in their study, there has been no consistent public gathering place hosted by YouTube to date. Despite this, the users that they interviewed overwhelmingly indicated that they did, in fact, actually feel a sense of community within the limited personal communication structures available on the platform (2009:41), and many of the vloggers I have been following make reference to that sense both in their videos and in the comments they make on others'. For instance, in early 2013, I noted a warm welcome to a new vlogger from some more established vloggers on bipolar disorder: "Congrats on your first video and a warm welcome to the community of uploaders! Good video to start with, now we know a bit about you we can look forward to hearing more from you. (when you have time!)." She fosters the sense of community by affirming the value of the new vlogger's contribution, encouraging more contributions. Another frequent vlogger offers, "good vlog buddy :)."[29]

Vloggers also affirm community by making videos directly addressing questions or comments from audience members. Some users post question and answer videos in which they post address comments and emails. Others do request videos, which are dedicated to a particular topic suggested by a viewer. SuperCrazylady21 has obliged several requests to talk about her experience with having an eating disorder and dating,[30] what she wants from life,[31] and how she does her makeup.[32] Vloggers create shout-out videos, in which a particular person or group is named and talked about as a form of recognition. One user created an entire text-only video, set to music, that lists the usernames of twenty-six vloggers who talk about mental illness.[33] Users give shout-outs to their audiences as well, showing their appreciation that people are watching and responding to their work.

Function 3: Promoting Self-Efficacy and Healing

Learning information about the disorder and forming and participating in a community focused on that disorder can be ways of promoting self-efficacy and healing. By becoming more knowledgeable and sharing that knowledge and making themselves available to facilitate community activity, they may feel further empowered and in control of their disorder. As anthropologist Michael Jackson tells us, "Storytelling [is] a vital human strategy for sustaining a sense of agency in the face of disempowering circumstances" (2002:15), and at the very minimum, vloggers do have control of the narrative of their disorder.

Some users explicitly state that they are using YouTube as a form of therapy. The belief that narrative can be a positive form of treatment for mental illness also exists in the institutional biomedical health system from Freud to modern day psychology. The belief in the healing power of narrative is articulated in different times and ways. User MM01 posted a particularly emotional video describing a troubling event and ended it with, "all right, I got some demons out on that one. That's good."[34] What is more, keeping narratives about mental illness "in"—that is, not telling their stories—is perceived as detrimental. Proof of its effectiveness is whether the individual telling the narrative feels better after having told the story, or whether the listener feels better after having heard it, and anecdotal evidence suggests that this happens frequently enough for vloggers to want to continue their work. In narrating positive steps toward managing their illnesses, they are positioning themselves to both the audience and themselves as agents of their own healing.

Function 4: Mitigating Stigma

Finally, many of the vloggers articulate that they are telling their stories in the publicly accessible forum of YouTube in order to combat stigma. Everythingamelia says:

> something that really, really bothers me about mental illness is the stigma that's attached to it and the prejudice, and this idea that people shouldn't talk about it. I've had people tell me that I shouldn't tell people that I'm bipolar because they're going to judge me for it and they're not going to want to be my friend or have a part in my life.[35]

On YouTube, fighting the stigma of bipolar disorder has taken many forms, from the vloggers who dedicate most or all of their channels to discussing it to those for whom a bipolar "outing" video is a one- or two-time occurrence.

Minor YouTube celebrities like model and actress Liz Katz,[36] fashion maven HelloHannahCho,[37] and anime reviewer HappiLeeErin[38] have all posted videos revealing their experience with bipolar disorder in the context of channels largely dedicated to a different topic. The common sentiment is that in order to fight the stigma of mental illness, people should talk about their own experience with it, which will help correct misconceptions and negative responses from those who do not have mental illness.

Stigma exists, according to sociologist Erving Goffman (1986:4), in the "relationship between attribute and stereotype." The stereotypes associated with mental illness in general and bipolar disorder in specific abound. In a discussion on stigma and illness, folklorist Sheila Bock observes that:

> it is worthwhile to draw a distinction between stigma (the effect) and stigmatizing storylines (the naturalized connection between label and stereotype that lays the foundation for the effect). . . . I use the term storylines deliberately here: negative attributes associated with diabetes become connected to certain emplotments that are, in turn, projected onto the life stories of the stigmatized. (2012:159)

Bock continues, "Stigmatizing storylines occur when stereotypical categories overdetermine individual identities" (159). Some vloggers directly address these storylines.

Probably the strongest negative stereotype is that people with bipolar disorder, and mental illness in general, are inherently dangerous and even violent. Desa Kroma dispels that idea with a combination of personal experience and statistics about mental illness. Regarding her personal experience, she writes:

> Being bipolar doesn't make me violent, I've never thrown my glass down at a bar and gotten into a fight, you know what I'm saying? I've never had like crazy road rage where I wanted to kill somebody else I was so upset. When I'm manic, I'm usually super happy, or I'm like super agitated, but not in like a violent way . . . and I do get destructive and I am a little bit out of my mind, but I'm not like physically assaulting people or anything like that, I don't turn into a completely different person.[39]

Vloggers also commonly attempt to dispel the stereotype about what people with bipolar disorder look like. One vlogger fielded a comment suggesting that mental illness should inherently impede her ability to dress and groom herself.[40] An outward identifier of a stigmatized condition provides onlookers with a frame that will aid them in placing the individual into a category (see Goffman 1986); apparently, a wild-eyed, unwashed person with unkempt hair in some ways is less dangerous than one who is neatly dressed and groomed but has the same condition.

Good mental health is also associated with attractiveness, which to some may hide the stigmatized condition. One woman's video prompted the comment, "It always shocks me to see someone so pretty suffer from this type of condition."[41] The opposite is the stereotype that an extremely attractive person, particularly a woman, *must* be crazy, otherwise she is "too good to be true," as in this comment on a vlog: "Why do the beautiful ones always have to be bat shit crazy."[42]

The discord between outward state (which is "creditable") and internal state (which is "discreditable") can lend people with mental illness the ability to "pass" for someone without it (Goffman 1986: 41–42). The analogy to being in or out of the closet about homosexuality is frequently used in the bipolar vlogging community, and Desa Kroma takes the analogy further:

> People were wary of . . . homosexuals. But then, what happens? You meet a gay person. Who's openly gay. And you're like, "This is a cool normal person. They're a nice person. They're a good person. I don't need to be afraid of homosexuality. They're not out to get me." And I think the more people are start to be out and open about it, the more people are like, 'Oh, okay'. . . . It became less taboo because people were open and the openness inspired more openness which inspired more acceptance.[43]

Different levels of severity of the illness have different kinds of stigma. The severity of illness may be reflected in the amounts and kinds of medications that a person is prescribed, and one user agrees with Desa Kroma, saying that in her experience, medication for depression has become accepted and commonplace. "But you tell somebody that you're on a mood stabilizer [like lithium] and holy fucking shit, it's like the sky opens up and you are an evil, evil person, and it's like you have cancer or AIDS or something."[44]

One common topic of discussion is the stigma of taking medication. The stigma here suggests that mental illness is a weakness of character or failure of willpower and should be controllable without artificial help. Arguments also abound about the overprescription of medication, the profit interests of the pharmaceutical industry, the long-term effects of medication on the population and ecosystem, and the lack of knowledge about how medication actually works. Even some who do take medication—and appreciate how medication has changed the course of their disorder—say that, given the choice, they would prefer to not have to take it. Some individuals explain the circumstances that prompted them to begin taking medication, as in the following from the user named ManicDepressive Michelle:

> For me I learned how to cope without meds for a really long time. Probably about 15 years. But in my personal experience life just gets in the way. Coping is not enough. I needed a job. I had a daughter. I needed to pay my bills and stop getting fired. I could no longer step away from a stressful situation to calm myself down. I needed to face the stress head on because I had no choice. To stop scaring my daughter because I was yelling at her and pushing her to the ground. (I'm not proud of that.) It's awesome that some people can live without, I tried for a REALLY long time.[45]

A trend that I have noticed in informal contexts (for example, my Facebook feed) is advocacy statements that compare mental illness to diseases like cancer or diabetes. This sentiment is echoed in the many of the vlogs I follow. This normalizing of the biomedical model can, in turn, stigmatize nonbiomedical perspectives. One vlogger is also a public speaker sharing his perspective that bipolar disorder is not a disease, but a "spiritual awakening." I combed through many of his videos, curious about what backlash he might encounter; his videos seemed (meticulously) free of negative comments, despite the significant number of thumbs down some of them receive. I did see one negative comment, but it was deleted between the time I started writing this paragraph to when I went back to find the username of the person who posted. The deleted comment was simple: "CULT."[46]

Many of the vloggers in my study articulate that by telling their story of their experience with mental illness, they are rejecting the notion that mental illness is a condition deserving of stigmatization. As sociologists Bruce Link and Jo Phelan theorize, one of the critical components of stigma is the imposition of a line between an "us" and a "them," or the "normal" and the "crazy," and how that interacts with power structures that allow the stigmatized persons to be treated as lesser than those without the stigmatized condition (2001:367). Many of these vloggers are working to position themselves to audience members, both to people who do not have mental illness and want to learn more about it, and to people who do have mental illness and are seeking strategies to deal with it, on both sides of that line—both a "them," and an "us," or just an ordinary person who happens to have mental illness. Desa Kroma summarizes: "This is why I think doing videos [about bipolar disorder] is important for me, just for my own peace of mind, because I think it's that next step that kind of needs to happen, people need to be talking about it in this sort of way, this being frank about it. . . . I'm just a normal person."[47]

Conclusion

When I came across these communities of vloggers talking about their personal experience with bipolar disorder, I could see hints of a "set of rules, a system of communication, a grammar, in which the relationships between the attributes of verbal messages and the sociocultural reality are in constant interplay," as Dan Ben-Amos and Kenneth Goldstein state in their introduction to their seminal collection of essays in ethnography of communication (1975:3). The four functions that I theorize are by no means the only functions possible within this communicative medium, but in all—providing information, forming community, promoting self-efficacy and healing, and mitigating stigma—were by far the most common, and while not all of them were present in every discrete vlog or every vlog channel, every vlog I followed could be said to serve at least one of these functions.

Realistically, for every vlogger who is active in my study, there are probably ten whose channels have fallen into disuse. Videos appear and disappear; channels are put up and taken down. One vlogger whose videos remain available has not had any activity on her channel for the past six years. However, new voices are continually adding themselves to the conversation. Many of the vloggers in my study articulate their appreciation for the platform of YouTube. This freedom does come with a price, though; there can be negative voices and negative consequences for posting. However, the vloggers who record and post their videos generally seem to believe that by doing so, they will be heard, and being heard will be good for them as well as their cause. The act of publicly sharing stories about personal experience with mental illness may, in fact, help decrease its stigma, because only when the private is made known can the public make meaning of the experience, too. The vloggers in my study, as storytellers of their lives, are putting a face to mental illness—an ordinary, everyday face.

Notes

1. This chapter is excerpted and modified from my dissertation titled *Narrative, Online Community, and Health Belief Systems: The Forms and Functions of YouTube Vlogs on Bipolar Disorder*, defended in the spring of 2014 at the University of Missouri. My thanks to Trevor

Blank, Andrea Kitta, Claire Schmidt, Elaine Lawless, and the vloggers whose comments helped shape this work.

2. Desa Kroma is a username created by this individual. She has given her permission to be quoted but requested that her real name not be revealed. All of the vloggers whose quotes appear here have given their permission to be quoted in my research; all of the videos discussed herein are currently or have been publicly available on YouTube.

3. The *Diagnostic and Statistical Manual of Mental Disorders* (DSM-5) (2013), a standard fixture in medical contexts in the United States, lists several kinds of bipolar disorder, each with its own diagnostic criteria. The two main ones talked about in the videos of my study are bipolar I and bipolar II. Bipolar I is characterized by manic episodes, marked by feelings of extreme happiness, outgoingness, or irritability, and depressive episodes, marked by feelings of sadness, hopelessness, and loss of interest. Bipolar II contains similar depressive episodes, but the manic episodes are called hypomanic, which are episodes "not severe enough to cause marked impairment in social or occupational functioning or to necessitate hospitalization" (American Psychiatric Association 2013).

4. For example, celebrity "coming out" stories appear on the covers of popular magazines, like Catherine Zeta Jones's 2011 feature in *People* (Hammel and Baker 2011).

5. YouTube no longer lists the country of origin for its video creators, but it did when I began watching videos informally in 2007. Some vloggers mention their location in their videos. For some, my assertion that they are from North America is based on my observations of comments they have made and their speech patterns.

6. YouTube Help, "Watch Time Optimization Tips." https://support.google.com/youtube/answer/141805?hl=en (accessed August 15, 2014).

7. The 2014 iteration of YouTube shows viewers several running statistics immediately below the video being displayed. One is a tally of the approval rating for the video, measured by a viewer's click on the "thumbs up" icon, representing approval or support, or the "thumbs down" icon, representing disapproval or dislike of the video.

8. "Vlog" is a portmanteau of "video web log." It can be a noun or a verb; as a noun it can refer to an entire body of work or to an individual video, and as a verb it is the act of creating a vlog.

9. Internet scholar Michael Strangelove calls vlogging part of a "mass outpouring of confessional discourse" that is unique to this era, writing that "the combination of features such as global distribution, mass involvement (as diarists and audiences), malleability, and audience interaction within online diaries is unprecedented" (2010:68–72).

10. YouTube Help, "Comment Moderation." https://support.google.com/youtube/answer/111870?hl=en&rd=1 (accessed May 5, 2014).

11. Bipolar Disorder Nerd, "Goodbye Bipolar Blog—Channel Shut Down—Harassment." This video is not publicly available. YouTube video, 1:42, posted March 11, 2013, https://www.youtube.com/watch?v=j2hJdW494s4&feature=youtu.be.

12. rawsammi, "Mixed Episodes in Bipolar Disorder." YouTube video, 11:19, posted August 15, 2013, https://www.youtube.com/watch?v=GRFfCIUfFZk.

13. Information-sharing by vloggers on bipolar disorder is not limited to Western biomedical perspectives and interpretation of the illness. For example, one user's channel is

dedicated to the idea that bipolar disorder is not a medical crisis, but a spiritual one. His narratives position himself at odds with the medical community and his own family and friends in his response to his disorder.

14. Desa Kroma, "Dealing with Hypomania," YouTube video, 15:00, posted April 7, 2014, https://www.youtube.com/watch?v=kuKuLBHdDXY&list=UUYZBoIq_GqXgNQh5M x36ECQ.

15. bipolardiscussions, "Risperdal Review (warning)," YouTube video, 3:49, posted August 24, 2012. https://www.youtube.com/watch?v=sdwwmO3zBeA.

16. bipolardiscussions, "Resperidol user review," YouTube video, 11:02, posted October 5, 2013. https://www.youtube.com/watch?v=t5ClUnj8Oik.

17. Ibid.

18. I owe this observation to a vlogger who did not wish her vlogs to be included in this chapter.

19. everythingamelia, "Everything Bipolar: MY STORY. The beginning of my battle against bipolar disorder," YouTube video, 14:00, posted December 9, 2011. http://www.you tube.com/watch?v=ENivdRZkmsA.

20. bipolarISme, "BIPOLAR DISORDER: My Story," YouTube video, 3:04, posted May 29, 2013. http://www.youtube.com/watch?v=jVWfARuhsq8.

21. SuperTuber2009, "My Bipolar Story," YouTube video, 3:33, posted July 16, 2009. http://www.youtube.com/watch?v=IEReHH1Kfwk&feature=related.

22. This video has been made private by the user, but she did give permission for me to quote her in my research before she took the video down.

23. This video has been made private by the user, but she did give permission for me to quote her in my research before she took the video down.

24. Comment on SuperCrazylady21, "I Have Schizoaffective Disorder." https://www.you tube.com/watch?v=KJj3S4dIexU.

25. rawsammi, "Am I Credible?," YouTube video, 7:16, posted June 2, 2013. https://www .youtube.com/watch?v=KnMb_GqvAeM.

26. SuperCrazylady21, "I'm a 'fake,'" YouTube video, 4:14. posted July 28, 2013. https://www.youtube.com/watch?v=oSJub81E3xA. SuperCrazylady21 had, at one point, been diagnosed with bipolar disorder, which was how I found her; her diagnosis was changed to schizoaffective disorder, which, according to the Mayo Clinic online, "is a condition in which a person experiences a combination of schizophrenia symptoms—such as hallucinations or delusions—and mood disorder symptoms, such as mania or depression." http://www.mayoclinic.org/diseases-conditions/schizoaffective-disorder/basics/definition/con -20029221 (accessed August 21, 2014).

27. SuperCrazylady21, "I Have Schizoaffective Disorder," YouTube video, 3:01, posted July 26, 2011. http://www.youtube.com/watch?v=KJj3S4dIexU.

28. Bipolar Disorder Nerd, "Being Bipolar/Manic Depression & First Doctor Visit," YouTube video, 17:28, posted July 10, 2012. https://www.youtube.com/watch?v=2QaBK_-78TM.

29. This video has been removed by the user.

30. SuperCrazylady21, "Dating & Eating Disorders (vid request)," YouTube video, 7:14, posted August 20, 2013. http://www.youtube.com/watch?v=oaHgD_khgjg.

31. SuperCrazylady21, "Vid Request::: What I Want out of Life," YouTube video, 3:24, posted June 8, 2013. http://www.youtube.com/watch?v=LyD7rVs5yCg.

32. SuperCrazylady21, "Make Up Tutorial ((vid Request))," YouTube video, 5:12, posted July 12, 2013. http://www.youtube.com/watch?v=QWVTg8FRb8U.

33. mooddisorderedmind, "More Great Vloggers :)," YouTube video, 1:39, August 22, 2013. http://www.youtube.com/watch?v=hG45AjBTiQY.

34. This video has been made private by the user, but she did give permission for me to quote her in my research before she took the video down.

35. everythingamelia, "Everything Bipolar: WHAT IS BIPOLAR DISORDER?" YouTube video, 10:41, posted November 30, 2011. https://www.youtube.com/watch?v=PtOWivLdfgs.

36. Liz Katz, "LIVING WITH BIPOLAR DISORDER (Manic Depression)," YouTube video, 10:26, posted January 22, 2014. https://www.youtube.com/watch?v=_Ne6GBqVDLU.

37. HelloHannahCho, "Bipolar & Me," YouTube video, 3:55, posted February 27, 2013. https://www.youtube.com/watch?v=VECRv58BG6k.

38. HappiLeeErin, "My Struggle with Bipolar Disorder," YouTube video, 15:33, posted June 9, 2013. https://www.youtube.com/watch?v=HKtOUNLnS88.

39. Desa Kroma, "Myths and Fears about Mental Illness," YouTube video, 8:27, posted November 22, 2013. http://www.youtube.com/watch?v=FLPY-KMqPp4.

40. reshmecka, "mental illness," YouTube video, 6:25, posted November 15, 2006. https://www.youtube.com/watch?v=fNZfPNMffzA.

41. Comment on HappiLeeErin, "My Struggle with Bipolar Disorder—YouTube." https://www.youtube.com/watch?v=HKtOUNLnS88.

42. Comment on rawsammi, "My Experience With Mania, Bipolar Disorder." https://www.youtube.com/watch?v=do3Fc684LBs.

43. Desa Kroma, "Stigma?? (Mental Illness)," YouTube video, 11:12, posted December 17, 2013. http://www.youtube.com/watch?v=u8lBfM7TCpU.

44. This video has been removed.

45. Comment on bipolardiscussions, "I'm bipolar and I don't take meds." http://www.youtube.com/watch?v=bpfDpGG3R68.

46. bipolarorwakingup, "23. Healing Bipolar Disorder—Moving Beyond NORMAL," YouTube, October 18, 2013. http://www.youtube.com/watch?v=A_3K2afvXvM.

47. Desa Kroma, "Stigma?? (Mental Illness)," YouTube video, 11:12, posted December 17, 2013. http://www.youtube.com/watch?v=u8lBfM7TCpU.

References

American Psychiatric Association. 2013. "Bipolar and Related Disorders." In *Diagnostic and Statistical Manual of Mental Disorders* (DSM-5). Washington, DC: American Psychiatric Association.

Bamberg, Michael G. W. 1997. "Positioning between Structure and Performance." *Journal of Narrative and Life History* 7 (1–4):335–42.

———. 2005. "Narrative Discourse and Identities." In *Narratology beyond Literary Criticism: Mediality Disciplinarity, Narratologia 6*, ed. Jan Christoph Meister, Tom Kindt, and Wilhelm Schernus, 213–37. Berlin: Walter de Gruyter.

Ben-Amos, Dan, and Kenneth S. Goldstein. 1975. "Introduction." In *Folklore: Performance and Communication*, ed. Dan Ben-Amos and Kenneth Goldstein, 1–7. Berlin: Walter de Gruyter.

Blank, Trevor J. 2013. "Hybridizing Folk Culture: Toward a Theory of New Media and Vernacular Discourse." *Western Folklore* 72 (2):105–30.

Bock, Sheila. 2012. "Contextualization, Reflexivity, and the Study of Diabetes-Related Stigma." *Journal of Folklore Research* 49 (2):153–78.

Bohmer, Carol, and Amy Shuman. 2008. *Rejecting Refugees: Political Asylum in the 21st Century*. London: Routledge.

Buccitelli, Anthony Bak. 2012. "Performance 2.0: Observations toward a Theory of the Digital Performance of Folklore." In *Folk Culture in the Digital Age: The Emergent Dynamics of Human Interaction*, ed. Trevor J. Blank, 60–84. Logan: Utah State University Press.

Burgess, Jean, and Joshua Green. 2009. *YouTube: Online Video and Participatory Culture*. Digital Media and Society Series. Cambridge, MA: Polity.

Goffman, Erving. 1986. *Stigma: Notes on the Management of Spoiled Identity*. New York: Simon and Schuster.

Goldstein, Diane E. 2000. "'When Ovaries Retire': Contrasting Women's Experiences with Feminist and Medical Models of Menopause." *Health*: 4 (3):309–23.

Hammel, Sara, and K. C. Baker. 2011. "Catherine Zeta Jones Bipolar Disorder: Her Private Struggle." *People* (April 14). http://www.people.com/people/article/0,,20481698,00.html.

Jackson, Michael. 2002. *The Politics of Storytelling: Violence, Transgression, and Intersubjectivity*. Copenhagen: Museum Tusculanum Press.

Kavoori, Anandam P. 2011. *Reading YouTube: The Critical Viewers Guide*. Digital Formations vol. 64. New York: Peter Lang.

Kirshenblatt-Gimblett, Barbara. 1996. "The Electronic Vernacular." In *Connected: Engagements with Media*, 21–65. Late Editions 3. Chicago, IL: University of Chicago Press.

Link, Bruce G., and Jo C. Phelan. 2001. "Conceptualizing Stigma." *Annual Review of Sociology* 27:363–85.

Rotman, Dana, Jennifer Golbeck, and Jennifer Preece. 2009. "The Community Is Where the Rapport Is—On Sense and Structure in the YouTube Community." In *Proceedings of the Fourth International Conference on Communities and Technologies*, ed. John M. Carroll, 41–50. New York: ACM Press.

Strangelove, Michael. 2010. *Watching YouTube: Extraordinary Videos by Ordinary People*. Digital Futures. Toronto: University of Toronto Press.

CHAPTER NINE

Tales from the Operating Theater: Medical Fetishism and the Taboo Performative Power of Erotic Medical Play

—London Brickley

In late December 2009, in an alley packed into the back corners of New York's West End, a man known simply as "The Physician" stands in the center of a room.[1] Surrounding him is an unfolding spread of the cool steel of a hospital cot and its matching industrial light. In the bed there lies a body. The body's face is occluded by an oxygen mask and the standing frame of the oversee-ing anesthesiologist. The skin of the body remains on display to the crowd—overly white beneath the industrial glow. The Physician calls to his assistant for the scalpel, which is presented to him alongside a bottle of iodine, cotton, and gauze. Snapping his own mask into place, The Physician takes the scalpel into his latex-covered fingers and prepares to cut. Those watching on do not know the body on the table. There is no glass separating the spectators from the operation, nor visitation hour restrictions. This is not a hospital, but a warehouse. The Physician is not a doctor, and the body on the table is not a patient. This is simply another night in the world of *medical fetishism*—a subculture whose participants find sexual eroticism in medical-related play, practices, procedures, roles, and aesthetics. The Physician, an active member of the medical fetish scene for over twenty-five years, had kindly invited me to join him and some of his medical enthusiast friends for an evening ware-house operation. This invite marked my thirty-first attended "live surgery" performance (a sort of medical fetish folk custom celebrating the days when operating rooms were called operating theaters and surgical procedures were performed in front of students and spectators).[2] As I watched The Physician's scalpel slice its way down the sternum of the anonymous torso with a steady hand, the mirror above the bed reflected the opening skin to its onlookers. Those in attendance knew the cut was only the shallowest of slices, meant for show, symbolism, and sensation, but the blood as it ran was bright and real.[3]

The impromptu night of operation was not the first I had attended, but it was during that particular live surgery, surrounded by the enraptured women and men on The Physician's guest list, that my casual flirtation with the scene transformed into my official descent into ethnographic work. This chapter is a select summation of my five years of formal folklore fieldwork among medical fetish communities, focusing primarily on both private parties and public medical clubs in the United States and the United Kingdom. Unlike the participant groups found within most traditional approaches to ethnographic research, the medical fetish community is not regionally (or even virtually) located in one place. Instead, a medical fetishist in the emic or cultural (as opposed to the psychiatric) use of the term is often a self-appointed identity by individuals who find erotic pleasure in objects and acts found in modern and historical medical practice. In order to create a sense of community, medical fetishists from all over the world have established conventions, night clubs, private gatherings, social networking sites, and online resources that cover a range of information from medical play advice, safety procedures, and links to specialty shops to purchase medical supplies. Out of this globalized community there has emerged a rich culture of art, fashion, and material; styles of performance; insider semantics; rituals; aesthetics; codes of conduct; and traditions.

Outside the walls of fetish participation, sexual fetish subcultures can contain difficult lifestyle choices for nonfetishists to understand. Traditionally, sexual fetishism was understood by psychiatric practices during the turn of the century as an "abnormal attraction" to objects or situations (see Krafft-Ebing 1965). Fetishists themselves, on the other hand, tend to view these regulating restrictions on human sexuality as an invisible line produced by a given culture's stigma and taboos. From the fetish culture's viewpoint, what the medical literature defines as normal sexuality (or what fetishists refer to as vanilla sex) is simply a blinder technique against, or disavowal from, the components of the human body, culture, history, psychology, and medicine that the majority of society doesn't want to acknowledge. In this way, from either side of the fetish insider/outsider divide, fetishism is more simply contextualized as a sexual or erotic interaction with concepts and objects that hold a stigmatized or taboo position in society. In the case of medical fetishism, the stigmas and taboos explored through erotic play are narrowed down to the often-silenced, forgotten, or ignored pieces of health care and its history.[4]

My ethnographic approach to the medical fetish community accepts fetishist or insider definitions of fetishism as a form of informed, erotic transgression. Furthermore, throughout this chapter I have intentionally chosen to respect and employ the emic use of the third-person singular "they" as the increasingly popular pronoun of choice among people who do not identify with the stark he/she gender binary divide—many of whom are members of the fetish community. With these terms in place, the particular content portion of the project presented here focuses on a specific selection of cultural components found within medical fetish practice in order to consider the ways in which medical play as an enacted taboo performance serves as a slanted mirror through which to view the traditionally stigmatized and silenced sides of Western medicine and health care.

Behind the Red Door: My Descent into the Literal Underground of Medical Play

I first came across the medical fetish community thirteen years ago in London, England, in a basement party of an industrial building just south of the Camden Lock. I could feel the heavy bass through the pavement as I wandered past the red door. It was well into the night and slices of the fluorescents from the nearby clubs made the rain look that much more wet. Just outside the door stood a woman. Expanding upwards of six feet on four-inch heels, she wore a tight white nursing dress of PVC that somehow both refracted and absorbed the light.[5] I watched her pull off the blue surgeon's mask from around her lips and light a cigarette. When she turned back inside and descended the stairs, I followed. Past the red door stretched red walls—not the deep burgundy of brothels and bohemian hotels, but the bright red of fresh oxygenated blood. If there were an official color of medical fetishism, it would be red. Throughout one medical scene after another, there are plenty of colors: the pale blue of masks, the industrial white of cotton and gauze, the slightly darkened sea foam green of scrubs, and the cold metallic tinge of steel. But among these pale imitations of pigment, the red is what pops— the blood, the signature cross, and more blood. True to medical fetish form, the red walls of the room created another sort of world in which the people glowed in undersaturated spectral hues against its backdrop.

The club, as I would later learn, was a relatively recent arrival to North London. The idea behind the nascent enterprise was to cater to the deviant and alternative subcultures that Camden Town had always embraced. The club's great experiment was to host different themed nights to give cultural subgroups a space to express themselves properly with fellow like-minded people. I had happened upon the night for the medical fetishists. This night— cleverly dubbed IntraVenus by the evening's hosts—set the visual precedence for the aesthetic that proved to be rather standard for the medical fetish scene. The dress code largely revolved around the staples: doctor scrubs, nurse uniforms, and standard issue hospital gowns. There were also the slightly less popular, but still often seen, options of straitjackets, full-body casts, and Milwaukee braces.[6] The room itself had been arranged into a makeshift trauma unit of sorts, the kind one might encounter after some unforeseen disaster required the emergency department to overflow into the neighboring high school gym. Shower curtains partitioned off sections for patient beds and exam rooms to simulate privacy, while other cots remained in the direct center of the room on platforms, serving as the operating theater for live surgical (play) procedures and performances. Around this main surgical display, private play continued on in a constant flow of motion and machines. Men and women wrapped in latex and cotton flurried about, applying oxygen masks, casts, catheters, stitches, saline injections, and IVs. Others just stood and watched on as scene doctors and nurses performed medical checkups with stethoscopes and thermometers or gynecological exams on vintage gynecological tables.

That night I watched. The fetish play world made me just another voyeur—not a particularly uncommon sight in the scene. I have always harbored a deep fascination for human sexology and was enthralled by this basement culture with its range of human expression. The world within these walls pulsed with an undercurrent of something dangerous and dark despite its vibrant hue. And so I came back—and kept coming back—until I could break away from my limited position as onlooker and speak, question, participate, and learn the elements of the eroticism of medicine and those who are compelled to seek it. I soon discovered that this bright and bloody world had much more in common with mainstream hospitals and healthcare systems than a casual observer might originally think. There was a method to this medical madness that wasn't so mad at all.

The Players: Taboo Transgressions of Power through Doctor/Patient[7] Role Play

"I challenge you to find a kid who has made it to their 10th birthday without having 'played doctor' at least once."
—twenty-four-year-old surgical fetishist

The most readily apparent components of medical fetish practices are the culture's surface aesthetics. How participants in the scene dress, along with the props and objects incorporated into the play, are the easiest for any observer to spot. Many of the time period choices in clothing and medical equipment in the scene are contemporary to modern medicine, although fetishist attendees of public medical-themed clubs may add a clubbing or fetish twist with adornments of PVC and rubber fabrics, corset inspired braces, and glow in the dark casts. Following behind the contemporary look, elements of Victorian and/or steampunk[8] aesthetics have become increasingly popular in the United States to incorporate into medical play.

In the case of clothing and time period selections, the choice of dress not only encapsulates an erotic aesthetic, but also dictates the designated role or position of the people involved. The most common roles found within medical fetish play are standard hospital fare: doctors, nurses, and hospital patients, although asylum patients, "mad scientists," and sadistic dentists also have their place. Taking on a dressed role during medical play can indicate a variety of affiliations with that position, from simply finding eroticism in the look and feel of medical scrubs all the way up to constructing a personal persona in the scene. Almost all participants identify with a given role for a reason, and most of those that do link it in some way to what a given role or position allows in terms of activities, implements, and above all else distribution of power. Who has the power in a scene is dependent on the other people participating. Doctors, surgeons, and mad scientists tend to have the highest levels of control, nurses and asylum staff have mid-levels of control (whereby they have power over patients, but often submit to doctors), while medical and psychiatric patients often enjoy acts of submission or positions of yielding power to medical professionals.

This hierarchal structure doesn't simply resemble historical and contemporary undercurrents of power distribution in generalized Western medical practice, but deliberately calls attention to it. Power play,[9] or role-play involving unequal power distribution, is a common element to the general fetish lifestyle in which Dominance and submission (D/s) and bondage and sadomasochism (BDSM) is a longstanding primary, but not exclusionary, component. Whereas many of the more generalized BDSM cultures have created their own power-defined roles with their own sets of guidelines (see Makai 2013), one of the draws for medical power players is the readily available cultural models provided by Western and East Asian health care, which position medical specialists and surgeons as the top level of command with little-to-no power granted to the patient over the trajectory of their own care. This model is often further supplemented in medical play by participants' personal experiences with power distribution among "real" healthcare systems and professionals. As Andy, a twenty-five-year-old medical patient player, explains:

[A patient] gives up control the second you enter the hospital. Plus you learn pretty quickly that you're a patient, not a person. . . . I was in and out of the hospital a lot as a kid. . . . I never really had control of my body. It would just fail on me sometimes. And then there were these doctors that kept saying things to my parents I didn't understand. They just kept telling me to do things or just doing them to me. They'd say, "put your arm out" and just take my blood or poke at me with something. I was looking out of my body but not all that attached to it. Between the constant needles and the IVs, I was just their pincushion medical experiment. I was powerless.

In an erotic re-creation of his childhood hospital stays, Andy's participation in the scene ranges from a variety of activities (play exams, bed restraints, and oxygen masks), but his top interests revolve around people and activities that can place him back "in a state of helpless submission" to the medical system. Andy's desire to take on the role of submissive patient is one of the most common in the scene, and it is particularly prevalent among players who had experienced "real" medical-related interactions that restricted patient agency and/or produced conflicting feelings in the patient over their lack of control.

The desire to submit and/or to seek out a submissive role in erotic play is one that many outside of fetish culture often have difficulty understanding. The important distinction between submission in the so-called vanilla (nonfetish) world and submission in the fetish world is that the core of fetish submission is paradoxically a form of empowerment. Power distribution in fetish practice is a simulacrum. Those in positions of dominance appear to control the actions of a scene, but it is the one in the submitting role who has set the boundaries and parameters of what the dominant role can do, as well as can "call the scene" (stop or end it) at any time. Freely submitting by choice to a situation that in circumstances outside of the fetish realm would take away agency thereby becomes a way of taking agency back through simulated play. Like Andy, many who do submit or take on the "helpless" role in medical play—be it consciously or instinctively—invoke the inequality of power and agency for patients' bodies, which are only able to reclaim power in a medical scenario when it is transformed through medical play.

The transfer of power is not always born from personal and contemporary medical experience, but can be historical as well. Historical, archetypal roles in the scene revive specific societal histories, which provide templates for grossly slanted power distributions between medical professionals and patient care. Like the players of contemporary medicine, historical players will usually hold a great deal of knowledge about the practices, tools, procedures, and the social or cultural climates of the time that they incorporate into their medical play. One of the more popular historical archetypes, asylum role-players, draws from the institutional side of medical practice, recalling a time in which variations of mental and/or physical health meant involuntary confinement in state-run sanatoriums.[10] Asylum play patients can often be found in the medical fetish scene bound in straitjackets, strapped to medical regulation beds, and receiving electroshock treatments. Connie, an asylum patient player who has a particular affection for institutions from the 1960s, often dwells on the horror of historical psychiatric practices of abuse and abandonment (see Scull 2007). On the level of role-based power play, Connie points to the apathy of the doctors and the isolated objectification of the patient. As she remarks, "Imagine being this person that no one wanted to deal with so they just lock you away. That thought makes my heartbeat pound. I can feel my insides screaming and there is no release." For Connie, playing the restricted and abandoned body in the scene helps her channel the history-born anxiety into an erotic and shared experience. If the experience is shared with others, then she can think about the profound isolation but know she is not actually powerless or alone.

In a (slightly) different historical variation of questionable power dynamics, Victorian-style play reenacts a time when "female hysteria" was treated,[11] in the more "extreme cases," with court-mandated hysterectomies and asylum stays, or in less severe cases, with clinical administrations of paroxysm (orgasm) by medical specialists.[12] Donned in Victorian nightgowns, corsets, and waist coasts, the Victorian hysteria players increase the dynamic of Victorian Doctor/hysterical patient play with intermittent "forced" orgasms and orgasm denial administered to patients by stoic, detached doctors with Hitachi wands.[13] Victoria, a hysteria fetishist and history professor from Boston, Massachusetts, describes her attraction to Victorian medical power play as "reliving the abuse and oppression of women's sexuality." The draw for her toward erotic reenactments is in the reclamation of the female body, in that "the 'play' part of Victorian play reinforces that although the repression of female sexuality is still a problem in modern medical practice, we have at least come far enough to play with that horrendous idea and make it our own." As with asylum-players, the concept of play is the key; the simulation reaffirms that it is not "real."

In a similar play of experimental medicine and explorations of the more controversial methods of early medical science, the final principle scene archetypes of the "mad scientist" and the "butcher" (or "Barber-surgeon")[14] stretches history back even further to the onset of the Enlightenment, retelling a story of a time when procedure, proof, and reason overcame human compassion, lore, and worth in the name of science. Likened in the scene to the archetypal split of the civilized "gentleman vampire" versus the bestial "primitive werewolf," mad scientists and butchers share a similar dichotomous, legendary intrigue. However, whereas the mad scientist is refined with his waistcoat and precision clockwork technology, performing delicate operations in a laboratory of electric, braided metals and neon glowing liquids, the butcher is coarse, wears a blood-soaked apron, and firmly believes in the soundness of heroic medicine[15]—hacking his way through bodies with rusty saws and ungloved hands. Variant incarnations of detached doctors in the scene, the mad scientist and butcher archetypes will often also incorporate an incidental form of sadism, treating the (willing but pretending not to be) subject of his/her experiments with either the maniacal glee of advancing medical and scientific progress or an indifference to suffering as a casualty of the process.

One of the more delightfully decadent mad scientists in New York, The Electrician (a close childhood friend of The Physician and always recognizable by his ever-present top hat), has set his living room up as a hybrid eighteenth- and nineteenth-century laboratory that is albeit rife with anachronisms. Complete with bottles and jars of iridescent liquids and murky oils, mid-eighteenth-century surgical tools, and rebuilt replicas of early electrical experiments, The Electrician's laboratory has housed some of the more lavish private play scenes in New York's medical fetish community. The type of play scenes found within its walls include any type of reenacted surgical or scientific procedure in practice between the beginning of the 1700s to the death of Nikola Tesla in 1943, with special emphasis on electrical play, including Tesla coils, shock therapy, and violet wands.[16]

When asked to encapsulate his passion for the mad scientist persona and play, The Electrician excitedly spoke about the power in electricity, the frailty of the human body, and the hubris of medical science to try and control the two, let alone pair them together. "The whole idea of the mad scientist," he explained, "is that he works with these uncontrollable elemental forces. It's life and death—and considering some of the crazy inventions of the time period, it was usually death. But death during that period is so romantic; Frankenstein, alchemy . . . if the scientist is just mad enough you can bring the dead back into a certain kind of life! It's the ultimate power—the power of gods." John, a "surgical butcher" out of Atlanta who goes by Gear-Locke in the scene, expands on the power in medical science play in more sadistic terms: "Medical science is not about the people; it's about advancement. You can do whatever you need—what you *want*—in the name of science. How twisted is that?" Using "For Science!" as his personal motto (a motto that is quite popular among many other medical science players), John enjoys masochistic patients that similarly enjoy fully submitting to his "medical experiments," many of which, for historical accuracy, include a good bit of pain.

Sadistic elements are not restricted only to historical play. Contemporary medical procedures have their own levels of inflicted pain, which depending on the patient's pain tolerance or limit, could be simply shots and needles to urethral sounding. As such, modern medical players in the scene looking to add sadistic elements benefit in much the same way as historical play by utilizing the template of roles, tools, and procedures provided by modern medical practices coupled with the culturally ordained power awarded to medical figures. Overall, based on participants' narrative accounts and my own observations, the historical or contemporary simulated accuracy in positional power, and medical indifference to that power, is often at the heart of medical role and power play. Regardless of which available archetype found within medical fetishism a participant may identify with and/or select to play, each role comes neatly packaged with a distinct level of power. These levels are far from arbitrary selections mandated by the community, but rather embrace, and in the process expose, the power structures inherent to both past and present systems of medical practice on positional, social, gendered, and humanitarian levels.

The Play: Taboo Transgressions of the Body, Boundaries, and Control

"There is nothing more vulnerable than letting things get past the barrier of skin."
—Twenty-one-year-old medical examiner and needle player

Selecting archetypal roles from the medical system in order to reenact them in medical play is only the first step of a two-part process. Whereas the first step is to cast the players in the scene, the second is to provide the physical content of the play or the procedures, practices, tools, and actions the set roles perform. Similar to the selected roles, the heart of the performances in medical play relies on a prescriptive cocktail of medicine's unspoken, stigmatized parts. Focusing largely on the patient's vulnerable position within the medical system, the performances become explorations of taboos surrounding the patient's body and boundaries, such as invasive procedures, inspections, and exams and the stigmatized emotions of humiliation, body-related shame, and control.

The specific forms medical play can take are as vast and varied as the past, present, and potential future of practices found in the medical field. If the object or procedure has been in any way used in medical practice, there is a good chance someone has incorporated it into medical play (although the more common a procedure is in medical practice, the more frequent it is in the scene). The top medical play procedure of choice is the standard medical inspection, or checkup. As one participant notes, medical play in general, and the checkup specifically, is, in essence, "playing doctor for adults." The difference is that playing doctor in the adult world carries with it a full-grown understanding of cultural expectations in regards to the body, privacy, and the taboo of being seen. For many inspection players, the erotic transgression comes from acknowledging and toying with the complex space of doctor/patient interaction during an exam. In speaking with participants in the scene, the general consensus of "looking at the body" is that the exams and procedures they had experienced outside of the medical fetish walls had always felt uncomfortable and detached. Many spoke of the inner conflict between the personal vulnerability they experienced during medical exams and the cultural expectation that medical professionals can, as one patient player states, "magically detach your parts or your disease into separate entities." He continues, "Maybe for the doctor they have 'seen it all before,' but for the patient, their body—and the inspection of that body— feels pretty damn personal."

Todd, an enthusiast of inspections because of their "dirty and wrong" quality, further describes the doctor's role in a patient's life as a "bizarre exception to privacy," playfully noting that "my mother always told me as a kid that there were 'special' places you didn't let anyone see—well anyone except the strange old guy in a white coat who gave me shots and candy." Checkups and other inspection-style play often explore the liminal line of this "bizarre exception" by playing with different scenarios a patient may experience during an exam, such as uncertainty of the doctor's intentions and professionalism, awkwardness or discomfort at being on display and inspected, and body-related shame that is subject to stigma and/or judgment from the inspector. Such exams may include an exaggerated physical—a medical procedure that requires a full-body workup of poking and prodding every inch and orifice—and gynecological exams in custom-ordered stirrup chairs. It is also typical for the participant playing the medical professional to affect a clinical detachment while looking too closely at parts of the body that hold cultural stigma—be it genitals, scars, birthmarks, or areas of body-related shame.

Invoking the clinical gaze of the stigmatized body in play allows participants to engage in a range of emotions, the most common of which are patient body-related shame and humiliation. In shame or humiliation scenarios, humiliation play seizes the opportunity to exploit the patients' lack of control over their body's physical situation in a way that makes the participant feel ashamed that they cannot control it. Incorporating the rather endless array of humiliation possibilities provided by the medical field into play scenarios involves tailoring the scene to the participant's personal areas of body stigma and shame. This could mean taking weight, height, and body mass index (BMI) measurements for participants who are anxious about their body at the doctor's office, taking the patient's temperature rectally instead of orally, inserting catheters to restrict bladder control, calling on a group of medical students (i.e., other participants in the scene) to apathetically observe the procedure, or engaging in "wet play" (stigmatized body fluids) where the application of catheters, supervised urination (part of a medical play checkup), diapering, enemas, or changing the menstrual pad/tampon of a restrained or immobilized patient, all reestablish the patient's helpless state and come with the looming threat that the doctor/nurse/orderly will see the results of the patient's bodily "waste"—material that is taboo, embarrassing, and "private."

Stephanie, a Los Angeles resident whose play includes both giving and receiving gynecological exams, discusses the unspoken erotic undercurrent of inspection that arises from complicated vulnerability:

> We have this idea that when things penetrate you it's either consensual sex or non-consensual [violation]. Then there's the doctor. You're consenting, *kind of*, because our society tells you that it's good for your health to make sure you get checked up; it's not supposed to be sexual. But then society also says genitals are sexual things, so it's kind of hard to detach yourself from your own body and sexuality just because you're in a doctor's office and because the social contract states that, yeah, the doctor has just inserted his hands and cold metal into your vagina while you're spread open for him, but both of you are supposed to pretend not to notice.

Elizabeth, another medical gynecological player from New York (who lives with her husband Steve and their custom modified gynecological chair from the 1930s) adds that "I still always get nervous going to my OBGYN. I was raised in a house where what my mother called 'lady parts' were something that women never talked about or let others see . . . [and so] I worried about how the doctor was 'judging' my body." Turning to her first play scene, "The first time I got in the chair," she says while pointing to the expanse of mustard yellow leather and metal parts in the corner of their living room, "I was as nervous as going to the doctor. I knew he was looking and judging, but the question of approval that I never got from the doctor was readily apparent with Steven. He *liked* looking. It still feels incredibly intimate every time."

The transformation of vulnerability into intimacy is a common component of play. The experience of facing body stigmas in medical exams is a general occurrence in health care, and yet, as participants in the scene see it, there are no outlets for patient anxiety and discomfort. Instead, the emotions and the need to speak about them churn and build until they are either repressed and ignored or finally expressed. For medical players, the play is the expression, channeled through the more tangible emotions of eroticism. The difference for the participant between body stigma experienced in "real" medical practice and in play comes down to the acknowledgment of intimate scenarios. In medical play, the recreated combination of clinical inspection and body stigma is often described by participants as a means of eroticizing medicine's aborted form of intimacy. As Allie, a nurse-player in the Atlanta scene observes: "if you are culturally encouraged since birth to regard something as private or shameful, showing or sharing that to another person feels incredibly intimate. However, if that intimacy isn't acknowledged or reciprocated it gets complicated." Inspection medical play showcases these emotional and situational complications, reenacting detached or dehumanizing procedures, but with the understanding that as a mutually agreed upon erotic experience, the intimacy is reciprocated.

In order to cut further into the tension of patient vulnerability and complicated intimacy, invasive play—medical procedures in which the body's orifices or barriers (skin and mucus membranes) are incised and/or penetrated—relies heavily on a range of medical tools and instruments (such as needles, scalpels, and speculums) and is often seen paired with inspections as an extra push into and through the body's vulnerable boundaries. Where inspections place the patient on passive full display, invasive elements engage all forms of sensory triggers to fully pull the patient into the game. During invasive play, tools and the environment become essential. Capitalizing on the inorganic severity of an exam room or operating theater, scenes are ideally carried out in as close to a medical facility simulated room as possible. To heighten the clinical austerity of the situation, as well as heighten the sensory experience, players prefer harsh light and sparse, inhospitable furnishings. In modern play, everything is sanitized and cold. The cold temperature and rigidity of metal and florescent light keep the patient alert and in a state of enforced vulnerability, which highlights the stark difference of the fragility of the body in contrast to industrial metals.

The medical tools used in invasive play are similarly selected for their aesthetic thrill and implied purpose, and/or are also selected for their ability to allow for the best sensation play. In scene explorations of patient vulnerability and/or medical sadism and power, participants tend to embrace the tools with the most torturous and terrifying aesthetics, use, and/or history. As one participant comments: "The more horrifying the device, the more I'm drawn to it. I can't believe some of those things were [and are] used on people as a cure. It's just bizarre and terrifying and that's what makes it hot." Such tools of terror may include bulb syringes, clamps, enema bags and hoses, speculums, forceps, electrical stimulants, prostate milking tools, urethral sounds, rectal thermometers, anal hooks, dental gags/braces, eye hooks, latex gloves, and Wartenberg pinwheels.[17] In time period play, medical implements can be modified further to take on the look and feel of the more severe objects of that particular medical era, including eye syringes, stomach pumps, tonsil clippers, electroshock equipment, and violet wands.

With the setting and tools at a participant's disposal,[18] invasive play explores all the medical inflictions a patient may endure, always testing the participant's comfort level, trust, and limits. Due to the nature of body invasion, this type of scene can involve elements referred to as "edge play" in fetish culture. Edge play, marked by the three B's—Blood, Blades, and Breath—are activities that could be harmful or dangerous if administered improperly. In the medical play world this includes (but is not limited to) sharp blades, scalpels, anesthesia, bloodletting, blood draws, and injections. To reduce the risk of danger, medical edge players are encouraged and/or enforced by the rules of the scene to take deliberate steps in educating themselves in order to acquire the necessary skills to achieve the medical play they desire to perform or experience. This could mean anything from finding medical mentors in the scene, taking EMT classes, or attending medical school. The more advanced training the participants of a scene have received, the more potential there is for safe edge play.

Alice, who has earned her certification in the "real" medical world of physician's assistant, employs her aptly named title at The Physician's abode as his resident PA. Her specialty is invasive needle play (injections and sutures) and anesthesiology. Alice's patients, when questioned about their experiences and desires toward incorporating invasive procedure play into their routine inspections, all expressed a preference for the increased taboo of passively allowing objects into the body. Many offered stories of early medical experiences that had felt "scary," "wrong," "confusing," or "uncomfortable" at the time, which became something they never talked about but acted out later. Others enjoyed the clinical lack of patient power (although, like the power role distribution, the patient also ultimately takes back agency in the position of *simulated* helplessness). As Alice explains, "The goal of invasive body play for the one receiving treatment is to feel violated and powerless." For a lot of invasive play, the patient finds an extra erotic thrill from being clinically

dehumanized to the extent that he/she is just another body to treat or diagnose—a viewpoint that many in the scene see as the current status of "real"
medical or hospital patients.

The overall idea behind invasive play is that once encased in the medical
system, things happen to the body and the patient is powerless to stop it. Following what Alice refers to as "the two-option rule," invasive play procedures
take on two distinct possible translations of a patient being "powerless," suc-
cinctly summarized by one participant as "to drug or not to drug." Harkening
back to the great divide in invasive procedures between a time in medical
practice when a patient's only option was painful, drugless surgery and the
onset offerings of surgical sedation, invasive-inclined participants performatively engage the murky ethical history of the advent of surgical anesthetics, prescription drugs, and the issues of consent, trials, and the side effects
that came with both (see Gawanda 2012; Kopp 1999). The resultant view of
the two-option rule is based on the lifestyle's understanding of the current
two options provided in a "real" medical invasive procedure: to remain alert
and experience all the pain of the body's procedural trauma, or to submit the
body and all of its conscious awareness over to the gloved, sanitized hands
of strangers. For the majority of invasive players (particularly historically
inclined players whose sadistic play relies on the time before anesthetics),
consciously experiencing invasive procedures and the fear, vulnerability, and
pain that accompanies them is the heart of the erotic process or thrill.

There are a select few extreme edge players in the scene that choose
instead to focus on the latter option, surrendering themselves over to the anxiety of abandoning the body to the hands of medical practice. In this form of
play, participants may employ over-the-counter drugs or (very) light aesthesia (with the patient's consent) in order to render the patient into an altered
and helpless state.[19] Although there is a known higher risk of harmful or fatal
complications, anesthesia players tend to take the looming threat as one more
part of their body that they can't control, ultimately regarding the risk as a
symbolic reflection of the concealed, always-lurking possibility of any medical procedure (death), as well as the ultimate form of medical vulnerability or
submissive power distribution. Amber, a practitioner of aesthesia edge play,
knows the safety risks that come with it, admitting: "Of course it's dangerous;
it's the most vulnerable your body can be. [Submitting to sedation] takes the
mind away from the body and leaves it all alone."

For Amber, the desire to seek out, submit, survive, and reclaim her understanding of the ultimate forms of patient vulnerability itches in her veins
as a pulsing need. It is a need that all medical fetish players know well—a
simmering blood bond that ties them together regardless of the physical

manifestations of their play. Drawing from my experience in the field, medical play revolving around power and patient control (or the lack of patient control) performs, under the guise of a thousand medical faces, a unified tale of culturally present body anxieties found within modern healthcare practices. The result of body-based power and control play, which simulate variant forms of vulnerability and increased helplessness, effectually capitalizes on the erotic fear of losing one or more systems of agency in an environment that the patient already feels they do not control. And yet—as found with the paradoxical power of submission in role and procedure play—submitting to simulations through erotic transgressive performances allows patients to explore and embrace stigmatized facets of the medical body in a controlled, reclaimed space.

In the end, the crux of all medical play comes back to power, and retaining power through choice, control, and consent while performing the perceived opposite of medical reality. For medical fetish players, Western medicine has, intermingled with its more positive qualities, a long and continuing history of uncomfortable ethics, painful procedures, and disquieting practices. Even in the twenty-first century, medical advancements have retained shards of medicine's heroic past. Slicing flesh and removing the pieces, sewing and stapling skin together, exposing, mutating, and eliminating cells through chemicals and radiation, and experimental human clinical trials all provide a richly infested ground for exploration of medical anxieties and body horror on which players in the scene have built their own operating theaters. Medical players celebrate the performance of the operating theater as the very pinnacle of medical anxiety. As the players see it, the "real" operating theater in medicine's history and its present is where patients go to surrender all and absolute control, undergo the most invasive of procedures, and cease to be anything but monitored flesh on a table. In a turnabout game, the medical players use the theater as a stage to enact and examine the medicine, while the transformation of complex emotions into erotic play provides tangible symbols with which to perform an exploratory surgery of the medical field's complications. As The Physician summates,

> There is power in medicine. We live, breathe, and die by it. It's an incredible power, but there are costs to that power. For wherever there is power there are also the powerless. It's easy to praise advancement and the prolonging of life. And that is worthy praise. But it's so much harder to peel back society's thriving dermal layer and examine the pockets of disease still infecting the bones. That's what we do here. We harness horror through desire to examine the examiners and play with the infested history of power.

Conclusion: Surgically Slicing the Silence

Perhaps it is all too easy for those outside of the medical fetish community—
or the "vanilla" folk—to look in from the outside and ask, "Why?" Medical
fetishists are quite used to this question, proposed to them by friends, family,
and strangers on a fairly regular basis. It is the questions of "why," the uneasi-
ness of outsiders with the practice of erotic medical play, and the hesitant
to outraged observers who find only nobility in the medical profession or
psychosis in fetish desire that keep the community fairly masked and seques-
tered. However, asking an individual medical fetishist "why" will get the infor-
mation-seeker nowhere. A fetishist participates in fetish play because they
must. The feeling of elation, eroticism, taboo transgression, fear, and arousal
are an innate part of their embodied experience. The feelings triggered by
"real" medical practices, histories, and taboos are not a choice, and participation in the medical fetish scene helps explore the excitement, terror, and need
in a safe, understanding space.

As a folkloristic approach to the community seeking simply to know the
culture and its people, my ethnographic approach never asked *why* seeking
instead narratives on how, in what way, for how long, and how it all makes
a participant feel, think, and play. In doing so, the stories, activities, rituals,
tools, and customs of erotic medical play inadvertently revealed a greater
"why" that was not an individual drive, but actions embedded in mass societal
and cultural concerns. Western medical practice has produced a long history
of power and procedure through a trail of body-bound stigmas and anxiety (Gawanda 2012; Hollingham 2013). There are problematic components
of mental and physical health care that have out of great necessity received
more widespread attention in recent years. And yet there are other elements
to health care that, due to a variety of stigma-bound silences, have not been as
universally examined in open mainstream channels. Politely overlooked and/
or silenced issues of inherent systems of power distribution and their effects
on patient positions and agency, cultural taboos over body functions and fluids, the invasive nature of medical care in contrast to cultural understandings
of "private parts," clinical objectification of patient bodies, and psychological
states of humiliation, body shame, and trust all have profound yet silenced
effects on patient vulnerability, comfort, and further physical and psychological development. Cultural taboos and social stigmas are by their very nature
things that maintain a culturally upheld understanding as subjects one must
not engage in or discuss. Eschewing the expectation that they will politely
ignore the uncomfortable sides of modern and historical health care, medical
fetishists delve right into the center of these complicated issues. The erotic

enjoyment and thrill of the transgression may be the reward, but the process is a full-body performance that engages; simulates; processes; reveals; and, for the briefest moments, reclaims power over the stigmatized body.

The women and men of the medical fetish community, stitched together from all regions of the world, do not exist outside of cultural and medical practice. Their bodies have "real" world medical histories and experiences, many of which shaped their attraction to, and participation in, the scene. A closer inspection of the community reveals that other than the derived eroticism of the medical procedures, there is nothing enacted or performed in medical play that hasn't been carried out in medical practice at some point. The transgressive performances of medical role-play are then intricately important contributions to the effort to combat health care and body stigma, providing outlets and voices willing to speak and explore. After all, fetish performances of repressed medical stigmas involve healthcare issues that have the potential to affect any individual body; the participants of the medical fetish community simply have the guts—and the willingness to play with them—to slice and break the silence.

Notes

1. Actual or scene names, ages, and locations of participants are provided with their full consent. Where such information is omitted, it is at the participant's request. All interviews and quotes were audio-recorded in the field with full participant knowledge and later transcribed. Particular acknowledgment of gratitude belongs to The Physician and his staff.

2. There is very little work available on the early history of the operating theater. The structures of the earliest theaters were often built in the shape of small amphitheaters. The table would be positioned in the center of the room so that surgical students and other spectators might watch and learn. This learning model has since fallen out of use, as conditions were dangerous and unsanitary (which mattered little at the time prior to germ theory and the push towards sterile and aseptic procedures). See Bishop (1995) and Hollingham (2013). Tales of spectator "splash zones" and surgical butchers who wore aprons instead of scrubs have become particularly popular ideas to draw from at medical nightclubs. One of the few remaining original operating theaters, The Old Operating Theater, located in London, now serves as a museum of surgical history and is a medical Mecca for historically inclined medical players. (The terminology of *theater* for the operating room continued for quite some time after the demise of the actual structure and is still in use in parts of the United Kingdom).

3. Surgical performances and/or play are only meant to simulate surgery while providing physical and psychological stimulation. Surgical play often involves the pretend act of cutting without actually breaking skin. There are blood players who will break skin, but not deep enough to cause lasting harm to the body. Those who participate in blood draws are

encouraged to comply with Risk Aware Consensual-Kink (RACK), a fetish lifestyle philosophy which condones potentially dangerous play provided all participating parties are aware and accepting of the risks and are consenting to the play.

4. Although the current prescriptive grammar crisis over the use of "health care vs. healthcare" elicits rather strong opinions among the term(s)' users, this chapter has no personal stake in the matter. Instead I have chosen to use "health care" throughout the chapter in keeping with the present standards of the *New England Journal of Medicine* on the sole basis that the journal is a particular favorite and most-often read publication among medical fetish participants.

5. PVC is a material plastic made from plastic polyvinyl chloride. PVC clothing is often a hybrid construction of multiple materials, typically combining polyvinyl chloride with polyester and polyurethane. As a result of the blend, the terms *PVC*, *Vinyl*, and *PU* can be used interchangeably, but *PVC* tends to be the more popular term among its wearers. The fabric itself has a distinct glossy plastic or "wetlook" that appeals to many medical players on both a sensory and aesthetic level.

6. Brace fetishes and/or brace wear can be found as a subset interest among medical fetish players, but also has grown into its own intricate community of individuals who exist separate from the medical fetish world. Brace wear can encompass a variety of erotic desire and play including the aesthetic of the brace, the feel of it, the experience of its wear, or the experience of watching someone else wear the brace, and so on. Alongside these nuanced complexities, the type of brace, its social and medical history, era of fashion, and used purpose all take on varying levels of interest for an individual and for its popularity among the community. The Milwaukee brace, specifically, is a back brace first designed in 1946 to treat a variety of spinal curvatures in children, including scoliosis. The brace is visually distinct, with its range extending from the pelvis all the way up to the base of the skull. Historically, each brace was custom tailored to the individual patient's body through a series of cast molds and was intended for long-term wear and prolonged mobility restriction. The history is one that lends itself well to the narratives of bondage, power, and control in medical fetish settings, and as such, the brace has a particular visibility in the scene.

7. With titles, positions, or archetypes enacted by fetish participants during power play, the roles that performatively control the scene and/or those in the Dominant position are capitalized, while those in the roles of submission are not. This is a written, semantic method of displaying power difference.

8. Steampunk, a subculture in its own right, re-envisions a Victorian futurism where steam power had remained the dominant technology (see Vandermeer 2011). For a folkloristic perspective on steampunk, see Hale (2013).

9. Fetish power play is the consenting distribution of power between two or more people in a play scene or "24/7" dynamic. Dominant or Top roles set and control the scene, while submissives or "bottoms" comply. The eroticism for power players on both sides is the simulated exploration of power hierarchies found in the "real" world and consensual submission to that structure.

10. There is an abundance of asylum lore among asylum fetishists, and many players have their own specific interests in particular institutions and/or psychiatric practices. The legend

of Pennhurst—a now-abandoned Pennsylvania asylum—was brought to public attention by NBC10 reporter Bill Baldini's 1968 exposé titled "Suffer the Little Children." The documentary footage, showing the interior of Pennhurst and an overcrowded population of abused, filthy, and neglected patients, was lauded as a civil rights catalyst for institutional care and is a medical fetish legend favorite (see preservepenhhurst.org).

11. "Female hysteria" was a widespread medical diagnosis in Western Europe, which reached both its height of popularity and decline in the nineteenth century (Micale 1995). The disease, to which all women were thought to be susceptible on account of the uterus and its potential to "wander" (become detached), float about, and cause "hysteria," became the diagnosis for symptoms of faintness, nervousness, restlessness, irritability, insomnia, loss of appetite (for food or sex), fluid retention, "heaviness in the abdomen," muscle spasm, shortness of breath, sexual desire, and a "tendency to cause trouble"(Maines 1998; see also Micale 1995).

12. Paroxysm was administered in designated physician offices, during which the doctor would manually stimulate the female's genitals until the paroxysm took place. This "muscle seizure" would appear to alleviate symptoms for a time, often requiring repeat doses of the procedure on a daily, weekly, or monthly basis depending on the patient. The practice was not seen as a sexual act but a tedious one that wreaked havoc on the physician's time and hand muscles. This eventually led to the invention of the vibrator, which manifested in its original form as a medical tool to ease the physician's labor (Maines 1998).

13. A Hitachi wand is an industrial strength vibrator ubiquitous to BDSM.

14. Prior to the professionalization of surgery, surgical procedures were performed by barbers rather than physicians. Barber surgery had an incredibly high mortality rate. See Gross (1996) and Himmelmann (2007).

15. *Heroic medicine* is a historical medical term applied to the experimental treatments and procedures popular up until the nineteenth century. As the lore goes, heroic medicine is named for the heroic feats that patients had to endure from dangerous and painful methods that killed more than they saved, such as bloodletting, toxic tonics, mercury wraps, and organ removal. See the work of Benjamin Rush (1746–1813), the "father of American psychiatry" and avid practitioner and documenting writer of heroic medical practice. An archive of Rush's work—and of other prominent heroic medical practitioners—is available through the *U.S. National Library of Medicine*'s Digital Collections Archive (http://collections.nlm.nih.gov/).

16. Violet wands are an electric stimulation tool designed by Nikola Tesla as a medical cure-all, which has been modified over time into its present state as a means of applying low current, high voltage, and high-frequency electricity to the skin (Carlson 2013; Tesla 1892). It is a medical fetish staple for those who enjoy steampunk aesthetics, mad scientist play, and/or historical "quack" medicine.

17. The Wartenberg pinwheel is a medical device used in medicine to test neurological function. The device itself resembles a miniature windmill with pointed spikes, which when rolled across the skin produces a reflex response from the nervous system, ranging from a tickling sensation all the way up to pinprick pain, depending on the applied pressure. Medical fetishists use the tool for its sensory and sadomasochistic experience.

18. Medical play equipment is easily purchased from specialty websites or bulk medical supply stores.

19. Drug-induced sensory deprivation in play scenes is considerably more rare, carries safety risks, and requires access, training, and knowledge of the drug. Crucial factors are what to give, how much, and what not to mix. However most play never reaches levels of sedation found in actual medical practice.

References

Ackerknecht, Erwin. 1982. *A Short History of Medicine*. Baltimore: Johns Hopkins University Press.

Apter, Emily. 1993. *Fetishism as Cultural Discourse*. Ithaca, NY: Cornell University Press.

Bancroft, John. 1997. *Researching Sexual Behavior: Methodological Issues*. Bloomington: Indiana University Press.

Bishop, William John. 1995. *The Early History of Surgery*. New York: Barnes & Noble.

Carlson, Bernard. 2013. *Tesla: Inventor of the Electrical Age*. Princeton, NJ: Princeton University Press.

Gawanda, Atul. 2012. "Two Hundred Years of Surgery." *New England Journal of Medicine* 366 (18):1716–23.

Gross, Dominik. 1996. "Arnold Schlegel (1850–1924) and the Agony of the Barber-Surgeons as a Profession." *Gesnerus—Swiss Journal of the History of Medicine and Sciences* 53 (1–2):67–86.

Hale, Matthew. 2013. "Airship Captains, Pith Helmets, & Other Assorted Brassy Bits: Steampunk Personas and Material-Semiotic Production." *New Directions in Folklore* 11 (1):3–34.

Himmelmann, Lars. 2007. "From Barber to Surgeon—The Process of Professionalization." *Svensk medicinhistorisk tidskrift* 11 (1):69–87.

Hollingham, Richard. 2013. *Blood and Guts: A History of Surgery*. New York: St. Martin's Press.

Kopp, Vincent. 1999. "Henry Knowles Beecher and the Development of Informed Consent in Anesthesia Research." *Anesthesiology* 90 (6):1756–65.

Krafft-Ebing, Richard Von. 1965. *Psychopathia Sexualis*. New York: Stein and Day.

Lederer, Susan. 2014. "The Challenges of Challenge Experiments." *New England Journal of Medicine* 371 (8):695–97.

Love, Brenda. 1994. *The Encyclopedia of Unusual Sex Practices*. New York: Barricade Books.

Maines, Rachel. 1998. *The Technology of Orgasm: "Hysteria," the Vibrator, and Women's Sexual Satisfaction*. Baltimore: The Johns Hopkins University Press.

Makai, Michael. 2013. *Domination & Submission: The BDSM Relationship Handbook*. Self-published, printed by CreateSpace Independent Publishing Platform.

McGrew, Roderick. 1985. *Encyclopedia of Medical History*. New York: McGraw Hill.

Micale, Mark. 1995. *Approaching Hysteria: Disease and Its Interpretations*. Princeton, NJ: Princeton University Press.

Scull, Andrew. 2007. *Madhouse: A Tragic Tale of Megalomania and Modern Medicine*. New Haven, CT: Yale University Press.

Tesla, Nikola. 1892. *Experiments with Alternate Currents of High Potential and High Frequency*. New York: W. J. Johnston.

Vandermeer, Jeff. 2011. *The Steampunk Bible*. New York: Harry N. Abrams.

CHAPTER TEN

Falling Out of Performance: Pragmatic Breakdown in Veterans' Storytelling

—Kristiana Willsey

Former army medic Curtis Feld was a soft-spoken,[1] introspective man, using his G.I. Bill benefits to study philosophy. Hearing of my research on narrative among veterans of Iraq and Afghanistan, he volunteered to be interviewed out of, he said, "thesis karma"—one scholar to another. When I asked him about the most dangerous thing he had done in his time as a medic, he began sorting through a handful of narrative abstracts, which he offered to me incredulously before finally settling on the time he received his combat medical badge:[2]

> Being twenty meters from someone and we're shootin at each other? I mean that's— (3 sec) Having a mortar land like six—like where that gray trash can is, and go off, but between you and that is what we call a T-wall? Um. Yeah, *that* can be scary. I felt the blast *through* the concrete wall. (1 sec) Umm. *Must*'ve been like a sixty mi—like a sixty millimeter mortar? (3 sec) Ahhhm, (3 sec) Glass shattering over a patient, me covering the patient? Y'know? (hits table) Gurney, uh, I remember taking these guys out to the helo? This is what (hits table) (2 sec) it's kinda *petty*, but (4 sec, indrawn breath, tapping table) They're all award friendly. I mean you have to *earn* it, I mean yeah, but it's just like (2 sec) I was taking patients out to a Black Hawk helicopter? We'd been receiving so many patients? And there were mortar rounds just falling. A-hahah-nd I (laughing) remember, pushing patients out on these gurneys, right a—what we call rickshaws. Not as a pejorative term to Asians, that used them but yeah so we're just (1 sec) Two-wheeled carriers and we're takin them out (hits table)

mortars are falling and the helicopters, they shouldn't be flying—I-it was a dust storm. See, the enemy . . . takes *advantage* of that. It-we can't *see*. Or we, *they* think we can't see *them*. (1 sec) And so uh (1 sec) bombs are falling and uh (1 sec) Yeah. I mean (2 sec) Uh (1 sec) Got knocked down a couple times, I mean, So. You said dangerous, not scared this time right? Okay yeah

(apparent digression, I make a move to ask a new question, he cuts in) So they gave some stupid award for that. (emphases added)

It isn't clear until the final line of the transcript that Curtis was trying to correct my question ("What's the most dangerous thing you ever did?") with a narrative about how he was distinguished for performing a difficult task under dangerous *conditions*. Since I didn't realize this, I thought he had abandoned the initial question and made a move to redirect the conversation. Curtis recognizes that he's about to lose the opportunity to talk about his receiving his combat medical badge and makes a final stab at narrative completion: "so they gave me some stupid award for that."

Curtis's story is a collection of sentence fragments, uncertain pauses, and descriptive passages with no clear plot or purpose. Yet as Bruce Jackson observes, "Sometimes what we think is a bungled story may seem bungled only because we don't understand the real story that is told . . . digressions and misdirections may not be errors so much as the enactment of another story entirely, one that is being told but one that we're not quite able to hear" (2007:32–33; see also Butler 1992, Mould 2012). Throughout this fragmented narrative, Curtis is actually still speaking to the subject of my question, talking around the time he loaded wounded soldiers into helicopters under fire, but he is responding to my word *dangerous*, as a judgment. Curtis is conflicted about his military career, proud of his awards yet embarrassed by them and not sure what they should mean to him as a civilian. The false starts, hesitations, frame-breaking, and other retreats from performance reflect his awareness of the simplified roles available to veterans—the hero, the victim, or the villain—that an uninformed audience like myself might bring to his narrative. Would telling this story be representing himself (perhaps misleadingly) as a "hero," or (per my question) as a "dangerous" man?

Curtis's story demonstrates how falling out of performance[3] can reflect the teller's unwillingness to take responsibility for a narrative that turns him/ her into a character that s/he can't comfortably "own"—sacrificing story to recuperate the connection that is the story's larger goal. This chapter reconsiders fragmented and broken narratives, not as eloquence attempted and fallen short of, but rather as strategic retreats from performance that key the emergent narrative as unfinished, thereby keeping the story out of circulation and maintaining control of the interpretation. Reframing retreats from performance as subtler or relative forms of success necessitates an inversion of Richard Bauman's now-classic definition of performance, "an assumption of responsibility to an audience for a display of communicative competence" (1977:11). Rather than treating performance as a choice assumed by the narrator, I focus instead on how the imposition of responsibility for a narrative may be deferred, negotiated, or otherwise managed.

For reasons that will be explored in this chapter, refusing or visibly avoiding storytelling is something civilians often associate with veterans and interpret this as evidence of the scars that war has left on the storyteller's psyche. The management of narrative—learning to select and edit stories appropriate for a given audience—is critical to avoiding the stigmatized identity of the traumatized veteran, who is either stubbornly silent or disturbingly voluble. Public exhortations to soldiers to tell their stories as a panacea for national wounds can put veterans in an impossible position: urging them to tell their war stories; necessitating the careful management of those stories for audiences increasingly disassociated from their wars; and then conflating any visible labor on those stories with the "spoiled identity" (Goffman 1959) of post-traumatic stress disorder (PTSD).[4]

The preference among scholars of oral literature has always been virtuosic performance, the "authentic or authoritative performance [which] occurs only at a certain point or in a certain respect. Other parts or aspects of the performance must be considered illustrative, or reportive, or even as oral *scholia*" (Hymes 2004:84; emphasis in original). Performance, for Dell Hymes, should not be a catch-all category, but a genre reserved for specific, heightened, specialized acts of artistic expression. This is hardly surprising; folklorists, especially, prefer to represent our interlocutors in ways they would want to own. When one visits a community of storytellers, one may ask to be directed to the artists, the "stars," those individuals whose contributions are recognized as the best, fullest, and most beautiful expressions of which their community is capable (Glassie 2006). In the course of my own research, my interlocutors often wondered why I wasn't talking to older veterans, whose stories were more impressive, more resolved, stories that had by now been deemed worthier of attention. But as Hayden White points out, "From the standpoint of an interest in narrative itself, a 'bad' narrative can tell us more about narrativity than a good one" (1981:14). My intention is not to expand the definition of virtuosic performance, but to shift attention to the subtler, fresher, more minimally realized stories, where the ongoing labor of the narrative is most visible, in order to emphasize how the current political climate encourages the conflation of emotionally or psychologically traumatic stories, and untellable stories, for which there is no appropriate social outlet.

Storytelling across a Divide

Narrativizing is seen as such a fundamental human practice that it is often taken for granted; we live so steeped in stories that we "ceaselessly substitute meaning for the straightforward copy of the events recounted" (Roland Barthes, quoted in Mitchell 1981:2). Because narrative can be a medium for empathy and understanding, "the practice is conflated with the process, and narrative, rather than particular strategies for its use, is claimed to be a curative, healing practice" (Shuman 2005:9). But narratives can also alienate, misrepresent, and create distance rather than cohesion. In an interview with NPR regarding his book *Redeployment* (2014), marine and memoirist Phil Klay reiterates that, too often, the stories that are told fall short of connecting veterans and civilians in meaningful ways: "What I really want—and I think what a lot of veterans want—is a sense of serious engagement with the wars . . . without resorting to the sort of comforting stories that allow us to tie a bow on the experience and move on."

Naturalizing the labor of narrative treats the sharing of experiences as a one-sided endeavor in which tellers hand off experiences like stable, static objects. But narratives are dialogic and interreliant—the experience being shared is the one created within the story, where teller and audience alike meet and vicariously relive the past. The naturalization of narrative obscures the responsibilities of the audience as co-authors (Duranti 1986) and puts the burden on veterans to both share their war experiences and simultaneously scaffold those experiences for an American public that (with the ongoing privatization of the military and the ever-shifting fronts of global warfare) is increasingly alienated from its military.

The space between military and civilian societies, in terms of contact and familiarity, is wider than it ever has been. A 2011 survey conducted by the Pew Research Center found that "while more than three-quarters of Americans over the age of 50 had an immediate family member who had served in the military, among Americans ages 18 to 29, the share was only a third" (Tavernise 2011). The gap lessens with age, but the affect was felt starkly by my own interlocutors (who largely fell into this eighteen-to-twenty-nine age range), using the G.I. Bill to complete their college degrees among peers who treated them as curiosities. The survey also found that veterans were more than twice as likely as civilians to have a child in the service; the postdraft military community has become increasingly insular.

This creeping compartmentalization leads to "a military far less connected to the rest of society, a condition that some academics have said might not bode well for the future of military-civilian relations (the military is run by civilians)" (Tavernise 2011). Rachel Maddow details the political history that has led to the ongoing alienation of the American public from the American military, noting that "the American public has been delicately insulated from the actuality of our ongoing wars. While a tiny fraction of men and women fighting our wars are deploying again and again, civilian life remains pretty much isolated in cost-free complacency" (2012:199). Veterans' narratives are often seen as the means to a cultural catharsis to atone for nationalistic sins, but the burden of facilitating understanding through narrative falls on veterans, not on an American public that (with an all-volunteer service and little day-to-day fallout from the country's drawn-out wars) is increasingly disengaged from its foreign policy.

Narratives Deferred and Denied

The drift of American military from the American public paradoxically puts greater pressure on veterans to tell their stories—to incorporate their unknowing fellow citizens into the embodied experience and political complexities of the wars being fought on their accounts—while at the same time creating a climate markedly unreceptive to veterans' stories. Former army sergeant Brad Fox, an aspiring filmmaker with a soft, surfer's drawl, explained to me that when he first returned from his deployment to Afghanistan, he wanted to be "open" when people questioned him about his combat experiences:

> I used to answer *all* those questions head-on, y'know cause I wanted to be like open—y'know like full disclosure, let people like, know about the experience kind of thing? [...] *Some*body that would, like, t-*talk* about it, as opposed to somebody that *wouldn't* talk about it?
> KW: Uh-huh.
> Ahh. So I *did* that at *first*, and then like ... I got weird reactions from people? Or like, it was very ... like, super vulnerable? Like doin that? And then like having somebody kind judge you with no frame of reference? And then like, givin you like these like, ((squirrelly)) eyes, and I was like, y'know maybe I shouldn't *do* this, like I should edit myself some more.

Brad clearly frames his early storytelling efforts in opposition to an imagined type: the silent, stoic warrior of previous generations, who refuses to tell his stories. Silences themselves can be telling (or misleading); as Tim Tangherlini writes in his ethnography of paramedics' storytelling, "If [. . .] they refuse to tell stories, they may be misinterpreted in another way; the audience may believe that the refusal is part of a representation of the difficulties of the profession" (1998:174). Silence can (unintentionally, perhaps incorrectly) signal to an audience that the story being sought is unspeakable or traumatic. Seeking to avoid such impressions, Brad wants to be seen as "somebody that would talk about it, as opposed to somebody that wouldn't talk about it." But he realizes quickly that in his earnest attempts to use storytelling as a means to close social gaps, he is in fact widening them—his audience is ill-equipped to interpret his experiences, and he is giving them too much information, or at least the wrong sort of information.

For veterans like Brad, learning *not* to tell certain stories is an accomplishment, a necessary skill to fit more smoothly into social situations. But the management of narrative for unentitled audiences blurs dangerously with the outright rejection of narrative, a denial of narrative's redemptive promises. There is a fine line between saying, "You can't understand this story" and "No one can understand any of my stories." Former marine corporal Dan Warner was a lanky, gregarious man who kept the helicopters flying during entry of the first wave of American troops into Afghanistan after 9/11. When I asked him what it looked like when someone tried, and failed, to tell a war story, he replied:

> I think when the story is a kind of therapy session? [. . .] Somebody who, is *telling* a story, and be*cause* of it they are *separating* themselves from the audience, I find it's very common. (1 sec) And I can think of one individual who *did* that, who's like . . . I had this experience, and you wouldn't understand, and it's like— And he's in a *room* full of veterans, and it's like, *yes* we *would*. Ah, and so there's, he's seeking to basically *exclude* himself. From the group, and (louder) if there's *any* environment where you could use this material
> KW: Mm-hmm.
> WARNER: Um. (1 sec) And, I think in *his* life, he had to *learn* how to *interpret* his storytelling. I-i-in a way, that could be received better. [. . .] How do I *understand* the world, how do I understand these experiences, how do I communicate what I understand *to* another person.

Dan denaturalizes narrative, breaking down the stages of emotional and intellectual labor that a virtuosic performance renders invisible. Knowing what stories to tell, and for what audiences, is not a natural or intuitive ability but a skill that must be learned, and Dan's anonymized reluctant narrator has stalled in the learning process. Dan emphasizes—and reiterates throughout the interview—that good stories are social. They can be dark and detailed, but they can't be painful or pointless because "when storytelling loses its dialogical dimensions it becomes not only self-referential and solipsistic, but pathological" (M. Jackson 2002:40). Dan offers me the example of a guy who sits there and talks like he's alone in the room, saying even to other vets, "You wouldn't understand." He sees this insistence on the privileged individuality of one's story, to the extent that it shuts down cooperative, empathetic sharing, as petty and irritating, even embarrassing to watch.

Particularly within military culture, with its emphases on masculinity and brotherhood, "emotion is an embarrassment. It marks an individual off from others; it signifies a failure of the social to encompass the subjective" (M. Jackson 2002:99). What Dan was describing is narrative that refuses to transcend the personal, and the first rule of telling stories is that something must be shared. Narratives that satisfy an audience are open, permitting the audience to leave the teller behind and read themselves into another's experience. Retreats from full commitment to the narrative—pauses, elaborations, and hesitant reframings—stem from an unwillingness to fully own the character-self, which has the practical effect of denying the audience the secondhand right to imagine themselves into that story and carry it on. Narratives that are knit too tightly to a teller's private world, that fail to fit smoothly into larger conversations, keep the focus on the teller and the telling, rather than the tale. Stories like Curtis's account of receiving his combat medical badge (being more frame than story) are not likely to be remembered and retold—which is, in fact, the point.

A narrative that breaks down presents itself to an audience as unfinished—literally and emotionally. It is less *repeatable*, in Hymes's third component of performativity (2004:85). A virtuosic performance is sometimes referred to as "owning it"—until the performer takes ownership of that performance, it can't be given away. It is the performance of entitlement, of the right to tell a story, which extends to the audience the right to take that story. As Amy Shuman notes, "a story survives by becoming another person's story," pinpointing the productive tension within the storytelling process: the transformation of narratives out of private experience is accomplished through a surrender of narrative control, a willingness to submit a personal experience to the collectivizing (perhaps simplifying, even bastardizing) impulse of an audience (2005:78). If the teller refuses to allow the audience an equal role in creating the narrative, the performance falters.

Incoherent, emotionally overdetermined stories are being keyed as private, not fit to travel. It was common in my fieldwork for vets to relate secondhand stories to me, crediting friends with full names and ranks—despite the fact that I had not and would not meet the original storyteller and that they knew I would be assigning pseudonyms to themselves and any individuals they named. Virtuosic secondhand stories were credited as a matter of course, while authors of narrative breakdowns were tactfully anonymized.[5] In the above example from Dan, he refers to the reluctant storyteller as "one individual who did that" and refers broadly to the narrative event rather than the content of the story. Taking one's story apart as it is told—repeatedly stepping back, breaking frame, elaborating, and second-guessing oneself—ensures that the story will not be sufficiently memorable to travel. Narratives package experience; they attach a point, a moral. Falling out of performance functions as a means to key the story as unfinished, a way of signaling, "Wait, let me keep this one to myself a little longer, this isn't ready yet."

Maintaining Control of the Narrative

Rather than a "breakthrough into performance" (Hymes 1975), Curtis Feld's would-be narrative is a series of retreats—he pulls back from the story repeatedly, and offers the point of it only as a hasty afterthought when it became clear that I had not picked up on his cues and was not asking the right questions to draw out his complicated feelings. Though withdrawing an emergent narrative may be strategic, this doesn't mean that breakdowns are willed or desired, or that a teller is not strenuously resisting first the act of telling the story and then the story's disintegration. It does mean, however, that there is something more significant at stake for the teller than his expectant, co-present audience: keeping control of the interpretation. Curtis spoke thoughtfully and in detail about the management of narratives for an audience and the troubling tendency of personal stories to travel beyond the teller's control. When I asked him what kinds of things journalists wanted him to talk about, Curtis laid out the complex problem of "telling it like it is" without "going too far." He had done several interviews for newspapers and had talked to enough reporters that he could say with confidence what they were looking for: a sound bite, something that reaffirmed the story they were constructing but had a different, arresting way of putting something:

> Something juicy, I guess? So, if I had to be graphic in explaining some of the
> events . . . that, I feel, would be going too far. You know? And, I don't really want

to do that. (1 sec) Um. (2 sec) That would be telling it how it *is*, but it wouldn't be … explaining … cause I don't like that aspect? To explain how I *felt* about it would be better for me, to, um … y'know, just kind of, dance around it? Y'know? So I-I-I kind of (2 sec) I-I-I don't (1 sec) I don't—uhh, penetrate into the past that I have, my memories of the past. Um. As graphically—if I was to be capable of it, as graphically as they appea-appear to me. It-it's just some visual memories and stuff like that.

Curtis frames his management of narrative not as a failure of language or of his own inability to transform his graphic memories into words, but as the maintenance of control and the audience's untrustworthy interpretations. He uses several spatial metaphors that construct memory and narrative as risky territory. He prefers to "dance around it," to walk the periphery of those memories, rather than "penetrating" that boundary and "going too far." Narrative literally *contains* memory, circumscribing the graphic, visual memories Curtis is talking around. The frequent pauses, hesitations, and self-corrections in this brief utterance testify to the consideration Curtis is giving his explanation, his concern that he might not be making himself understood. He repeatedly checks the connection we've established in the way one might tug on a rope to see if it will bear weight. "You know? You know?" he asks me again.

In this fragmented utterance, Curtis makes a distinction between sensation and evaluation—what he felt and "how [he] felt about it." Essentially, stories that offer sensation without evaluation put too much trust in their audiences. They function with the same ambiguity as raw images: "the photographer's intentions do not determine the meaning of the photograph, which will have its own career, blown by the whims and loyalties of the diverse communities that have use for it" (Sontag 2003:39). Those disseminating images are unable to control whether they will be read with horror, as instigation to social action, with a kind of primal fascination that inspires further violence, or even just with exhausted resignation that deadens through repeated exposure.

An evaluation that circles the darker memories and returns home leaves you with a narrative that is whole and resolved. A more vivid and uncertain account would leave the work of narrativizing, evaluating, and resolving to the listener. What Curtis is emphasizing in his preference for "dancing around it" is the discomfort of attempting to give an unknown audience a vicarious experience by getting graphic. Curtis is a reluctant narrator because to tell an especially detailed, sensory-rich narrative—"aesthetically redundant," to borrow Dorothy Noyes's (2011) phrase—would be to extend to that reporter (and his or her readership) a vicarious traumatic experience and perhaps give them the evocative equipment to read themselves into his memories and own that story. Juicy, arresting narratives have legs; they travel far from their original authors, out of their control. This is the risk that performance takes, what makes performance thrilling and dangerous—the knowledge that interpretation and reception are outside the artist's aegis, and whatever story passes from teller to audience does so by a profound act of trust. Curtis is unwilling to let an unknown, unauthorized audience do the dangerous work of making sense of sensation. Framed by the explanation that a potentially graphic description would be destined to be a sound bite, it becomes clearer that the critical issue is the ownership and management of Curtis's own story.

Skirting the edges of narrative, avoiding the graphic details that would offer a vicarious experience to audiences, is a strategy for the management of both story and self. The stories we tell allow us to step outside of experience and treat past selves as characters. As a projection of self becomes performance, it begins to be seen as "not-self." Linking theater to everyday life, Erving Goffman refers to this as "the power of dramatic scriptings to insulate performers from their parts" (quoted in Young 1986:104). This separation is productive, because the self-as-character is within the teller's grasp, miniaturized and manageable in a way that the teller's self is not (or, at least, was not in the moment of experience). Anthropologist Michael Jackson sums this up by saying, "storytelling is a coping strategy that involves making words stand for the world, and then, by manipulating them, changing one's *experience* of the world" (2002:18). As Jackson notes, the narrative is a product of the teller, under his or her control in a way that the world can never be. Through narrative, past events are remade and infused with order and significance, and previous selves can be reclaimed or discarded. For Curtis to grant audience members a vicarious look at those undescribed visual memories, rather than an account of how he felt about what he experienced, is to entrust them with the power to remake his world—not a responsibility one passes on lightly.

Traumatic and Untellable Narratives

Falling out of performance is a strategy for the management of identity, but it is also entangled with the image of the stigmatized reluctant narrator, the veteran who values individual control over social coherence. When the labor of narrative is taken for granted and stories are seen to extend privileged access to the teller's inner world, then the visible management of narrative— frame breaks, elaborations, hesitation, self-correction, and other markers of a narrative being carefully calibrated for an audience—appear unnecessary and overprotective, evidence of a pathological lack of faith in narrative's redemptive promises. Stories rendered untellable by context and audience are conflated with traumatic narrative, in which the narrator is emotionally or psychologically undone by the act of telling.

Diane Goldstein, describing the untellability of chaotic narratives—designating "*chaotic* for situations in which narrative confusion, fragmentation, or disorder is the result of traumatic, psychological, or intellectual challenge"—draws an important distinction between stories that become untellable because of context (the storytelling situation) and content in which the story can't be told because of "faulty memory, confusion, fragmentation, and an inability to articulate" (2012:181). Goldstein's consideration of chaotic narrative includes a parallel/additional dimension of *untellability*, determined by "audience expectations, newsworthiness, uniqueness, relevance, importance, and humor, but also—and perhaps just as centrally—appropriateness, contextualization, negotiation, mediation, and entitlement" (Goldstein and Shuman 2012:119). For the purpose of this chapter, I define tellability more narrowly, setting *traumatic* narrative—stories in which emotional or psychological distress fragments the performance—in opposition to *untellable* narrative, with untellability being used here to refer specifically to stories that context and audience have rendered inappropriate, irrelevant, or undesirable.

Goldstein's distinction between content and context parallels Dell Hymes's mutually dependent conditions for competent performance: "knowing what and knowing how; between knowledge, on the one hand, and motivation and identification, on the other" (2004:84–85). Hymes indicates that "knowing how" is a matter of "motivation and identification." As I have argued in this chapter, "motivation and identification" are closely linked; the willingness to tell a story is dependent upon identification with the story, upon the commitment to a particular version of self-as-character. When narratives split apart under the pressures of competing social requirements, it reflects unwillingness on the part of the teller to own texts that push the teller into an undesirable role. In conflating "knowing how" with "motivation and identification," Hymes treats *skill* as inseparable from *will*, an apparently trivial semantic issue that carries enormous significance for the politics of veterans' representation. Blurring the intellectual or emotional ability to verbalize a narrative and the social possibility of telling a story turns *untellable* narratives into *traumatic* ones. In other words, it becomes impossible to distinguish between stories that are not told because they are not socially appropriate and stories that are never told because the storyteller is emotionally or psychologically incapable of it. Without this distinction, tightly managed social strategy can be read as problematic pathology.

PTSD as Cultural Touchstone

If no distinction is made between stories that can't be told because a disengaged American public has made no place for them and stories that can't be told because returning soldiers are suffering from psychological disorders or injuries (depending on whether PTSD or the arguably less stigmatizing PTSI[6] is preferred), then the alienation many vets feel upon returning to their pre-war lives is treated as their own responsibility, part of their illness, and something else they must learn how to manage for the sake of their audiences. Many critics of the current treatment models for veterans argue that this is precisely what is wrong with how PTSD is diagnosed and treated.

In March 2012, an internal memo from the Madigan Army Medical Center outside of Tacoma, Washington, was leaked to the public. In the letter, a psychiatrist employed by the center asked whether certain cases could be labeled "personality disorders" rather than being diagnosed with PTSD, stating that "We have to ensure we are not just 'rubber stamping' a soldier with the diagnosis of PTSD.... We have to be good stewards of the tax-payer dollars" (Drummond 2012). There was justified public outcry over the exposure of financial interest affecting the medical care of veterans, but the more sensitive, unaddressed subtext was that medical categories are cultural, subjective, and political—that the labels we use to determine the impact of war are inventions of reality, not reflections of it. The story had to become "traumatized veterans are being denied the benefits they deserve," because if the story were instead "PTSD diagnoses are grounded in history, politics, and relationships, based on more than objective, measurable physiological symptoms," then the problem would be more complex than money—the problem would require a structural overhaul of how we understand and relate to our veterans.

A provocative article by David Dobbs (2009) in *Scientific American* argued that PTSD is overdiagnosed, in that the diagnosis is too fluid and subjective to have any real medical efficacy. PTSD, the critique holds, has become a catchall category that interprets depression, anxiety, and a variety of "healthy" responses to trauma as debilitating disorder, and consequently, they become so. As psychologist Richard McNally contends, "This has nothing to do with gaming or working the system or consciously looking for sympathy.... We all do this: We cast our lives in terms of narratives that help us understand them. A vet who's having a difficult life may remember a trauma, which may or may not have actually traumatized him, and everything makes sense" (quoted in Dobbs 2009). Arthur Kleinman, writing about individuals displaced by violence and seeking political asylum, calls the translation of their experiences into reductive terms for safety "another type of violation. Their memories of violation, their *trauma stories* become the currency with which they enter exchanges for physical resources" (1995:176). Veterans enter a similar arrangement; their stories are their "currency," even when no currency is changing hands.

None of these arguments deny that PTSD exists, but rather that the Veterans Affairs' treatment model is broken: if trauma is a necessary condition to receiving care, veterans will always be traumatized; there is no possibility for recovery because there is no existing vocabulary for it. Nevertheless, in a climate in which veterans often struggle to receive recognition and care for invisible injuries, claims that PTSD is overdiagnosed are fiercely contested by veterans who don't want the only terms they have to be threatened or discredited. To discuss the grounding of PTSD in cultural context comes dangerously close to saying, "It's all in your head" (though it's just the opposite).

Katherine Kim, a former active duty Army E4 (specialist), currently in the National Guard, describes the loneliness and depression she experienced when she returned from a peacekeeping mission in Kosovo and transitioned from full-time military life:

KATHERINE: My first semester at [her university], I am still shocked that I'm alive still. That first semester (2 sec) there were many times where I thought about jumping in front of a *semi*, jumping off a *bridge*—it was really hard. You can't go from an environment where you're sur*round*ed by people (1 sec) 24/7 and then I went to an environment where: I was completely alone, I had *no* support group, I was living in studio apartment by myself, didn't know a *damn* person in the area. [...]

Y'know, granted, I didn't see any combat. I didn't have to shoot my weapons. Umm but like, it was just *really*, really hard for me to come back, from an environment where I came home to somebody every day, I had somebody to eat lunch, dinner, breakfast with, *every* frickin day(.) y'know. [...]

My friend, [Fee's], like, "You might have PTSD," and I'm like (sarcastically) "Really? Really [Fee]? How'm I gonna have fuckin PTSD." She's like, "Well m— my boyfriend, my ex-boyfriend had broken up with me when I was in Kosovo, and she's like "Mmaybe that shit kinda fucked you up," I was like, "Really? Really?" And I mean I understand it's a relationship but I was like, "Whatever." But still. [...]

KW: Something I've heard more than once is that, you go from doing something really *important* all the time, to going and making—

KATHERINE: To doing *nothing*. Um. [Fee] said when she got back from Iraq she was just *angry* all the time.

Katherine jumps in to support my summation, that the abrupt shift from the significance of everyday work in the military to the "nothing" of life as a civilian is a common experience. She emphatically rejects her friend's suggested PTSD diagnosis but still feels that there is something there that merits her raising the conversation, without my prompting—her difficult transition was real, and she is confused and angry that there isn't a vocabulary to discuss it that doesn't make her appear as if she is claiming a "traumatized" identity she doesn't feel she deserves, compared to friends with more dangerous deployments.

Whether or not PTSD is in fact overdiagnosed (and whether that conversation helps vets or hurts them), the label certainly has more than medical significance. As anthropologist and VA researcher Erin Finley notes, "PTSD has the potential to become an identity as well as an illness, and this is not always to the good" (2011:172). Treating PTSD as an identity pushes it to serve a broader societal purpose: it shifts the accountability for violence away from individual soldiers and onto a faceless administration. The military occupies a liminal position between the powerful and the marginal, the official and the vernacular—soldiers are simultaneously an extension of their government and also free-thinking citizens constitutionally entitled to question their leaders' decisions. Representations of the military in popular media attempt to simplify these contradictory allegiances: soldiers can either be on the side of their government (heroes, if the public approves of the war and villains if they don't) or they can be on the side of a public that has disavowed an unpopular war. In order for civilians to simultaneously identify with their military and reject the decisions of their government, veterans become victims of politics, coerced into combat. PTSD exists in part to ritually recognize the proverb that "war is hell"—if not everyone who serves in wartime is traumatized by it, then the horrors of war are not being appropriately propitiated.

In some ways, a combat veteran without PTSD—who finds value in his war experiences rather than being crippled by them[7]— is a more troubling character to civilians. As Sebastian Junger, co-director of the award-winning documentary *Restrepo*,[8] writes,

> The idea that a psychologically healthy person could miss war seems an affront to the idea that war is evil. Combat is supposed to feel bad because undeniably bad things happen in it, but a fully human reaction is far more complex than that. If we civilians don't understand that complexity, we won't do a very good job of bringing these people home and making a place for them in our society. (Junger 2013)

The complex cultural grounding of PTSD parallels the blurring of boundaries between untellable narratives and specifically traumatic narratives. Veterans' narratives can break down due to emotional or psychological distress, or an uninformed and disengaged audience, or some combination of the above, but when most of the attention goes to the former, the problem becomes individual—or better still, seen as specific to the military's broken models for handling postservice adjustments. The story's flaws, like a PTSD diagnosis itself, becomes clinical, an individual's problem or a military problem, not a cultural problem that must be addressed beyond the confines of a therapist's office. It charges veterans with effortlessly orchestrating a kind of cultural catharsis, insisting that they not only tell their stories but also supply the necessary framework to make their stories coherent, and then stigmatizes the visible management of those stories.

If the cathartic, therapeutic function of narrative is foregrounded and essentialized, and storytelling itself is seen as synonymous with the work that storytelling accomplishes, then veterans must tell their stories, not just for their own individual recoveries, but as a proxy for the healing of a national audience. This expectation, coupled with the growing distance between the military and civilian populations, simultaneously *compels* and *destabilizes* veterans' narratives—and then interprets attempts to correct or control a story's collapse as a failure of the teller rather than of the audience. Narrative breakdowns act as part of a larger strategy for the presentation of self, but when narratives that are untellable for reasons that have as much to do with the audience as the teller become, by default, traumatic, it becomes the responsibility of the individual veteran to manage the threat of stigma. Like narratives, concepts of trauma, illness, and disability are socially determined and morally charged, acquiring coherence only when shared among members of a group. But in a medical search for origin stories, ever-advancing technologies for reading the body seek to locate illness within individuals, at a cellular or neurological level, rather than in the complex and intangible webs of interindividual relationships. To pin down definitions of health in isolation from the flux of culture is to leave the larger story untold, outside of the frame.

Transcription Key

[. . .]	short section omitted
[ ]	altered text (usually a name or place anonymized)

italics	stressed words or syllables
?	rising intonation at the end of an utterance
.	falling intonation, closing an utterance
,	pause
—	interruption, including self-correction
(sec)	longer pause, indicated with the number of seconds
((xx))	uncertain hearing, indecipherable (possible word in parentheses)
CAPITALS	volume
. . .	searching, anticipatory pause
(xx)	description of scene, gestures, transcriber's notes

Notes

1. All names have been anonymized.

2. A transcription key is at the end of this chapter.

3. In military language, "fall out" is a command to leave a formation prior to being dismissed. My use of "falling out" is a gesture to this—a deliberate rather than involuntary move.

4. I have used PTSD throughout as an emic term—the complex burden of associations it carries for veterans is partly the problem that changing the term (reasserting the medical diagnosis) would address.

5. One of the ethical issues with ethnographic research is the way in which the writing and review process itself can contradict the management of identity within the communities studied. Anonymity had to be provided to all of my interlocutors regardless of their preferences, but true anonymity is next to impossible to ensure in a study of narrative because individuals are identifiable by the stories themselves—people know whose stories are whose, and when stories move, the original teller is named. Not only am I breaking the rules by sharing these partially withdrawn narratives, but by anonymizing all my participants, I've equated skillful storytellers who fully own their performances with traumatized ones who don't, at least yet.

6. Post-Traumatic Stress Injury.

7. The growing body of research on "post traumatic growth" (see Calhoun and Tedeschi 2013; Weiss and Berger 2010) was exciting to some of my interlocutors as an alternative to the victimizing language of PTSD. But psychiatrists and mental health specialists are cautious, finding that the army's Master Resilience Trainer course, designed to test and instill "mental toughness," was implemented too quickly and without enough evidence that positive psychology would be effective against the sudden and severe stresses of combat (Rendon 2012).

8. *Restrepo* (2010) is a documentary directed and produced by journalist Sebastian Junger and the late photojournalist Tim Hetherington, recounting the experiences of the

2nd Platoon, B Company, 2nd Battalion, 503rd Infantry Regiment, 173rd Airborne Brigade Combat Team of the army during a fifteen-month deployment in Afghanistan's Korangal Valley. The film is named for Private First Class Juan Restrepo, killed in action early in the campaign, as well as for the outpost that the platoon constructed and named in his memory.

References

Bauman, Richard. 1977. *Verbal Art as Performance*. Long Grove, IL: Waveland Press.

Butler, Gary. 1992. "Indexicality, Authority, and Communication in Traditional 'Narrative Discourse.'" *Journal of American Folklore* 105 (415):34–56.

Calhoun, Lawrence, and Richard Tedeschi. 2013. *Posttraumatic Growth in Clinical Practice*. New York: Routledge.

Dobbs, David. 2009. "Soldiers' Stress: What Doctors Get Wrong About PTSD." *Scientific American* (April). http://www.scientificamerican.com/article/post-traumatic-stress-trap/.

Drummond, Kate. 2012. "Army Wants PTSD Clinicians to Stop Screening for Fakers." *Wired .com* (April 23). http://www.wired.com/dangerroom/2012/04/army-ptsd-guidelines.

Duranti, Alessandro. 1986. "The Audience as Co-Author: An Introduction." *Text* 6:239–47.

Finley, Erin P. 2011. *Fields of Combat: Understanding PTSD among Veterans of Iraq and Afghanistan*. Ithaca, NY: Cornell University Press.

Goldstein, Diane, and Amy Shuman. 2012. "The Stigmatized Vernacular: Where Reflexivity Meets Untellability." *Journal of Folklore Research* 49 (2):113–26.

Glassie, Henry. 2006. *The Stars of Ballymenone*. Bloomington: Indiana University Press.

Goffman, Erving. 1959 [1956]. *The Presentation of Self in Everyday Life*. Garden City, NY: Doubleday Anchor Books.

Hymes, Dell. 1975. "Breakthrough into Performance." In *Folklore: Performance and Communication*, ed. Dan Ben-Amos and Kenneth S. Goldstein, 11–74. The Hague, Netherlands: Mouton.

———. 2004 [1981]. *In Vain I Tried to Tell You: Essays in Native American Ethnopoetics*. Lincoln: University of Nebraska Press.

Jackson, Bruce. 2007. *The Story Is True: The Art and Meaning of Telling Stories*. Philadelphia: Temple University Press.

Jackson, Michael. 2006 [2002]. *The Politics of Storytelling: Violence, Transgression, and Intersubjectivity*. Copenhagen: Museum Tusculanum Press.

Junger, Sebastian. 2011. "Why Would Anyone Miss War?" *New York Times* (July 17). http://www.nytimes.com/2011/07/17/opinion/sunday/17junger.html?_r=0.

Klay, Phil. 2014. "Reminder from a Marine: Civilians and Veterans Share Ownership of War." Interview on *National Public Radio*, Morning Edition (March 6). http://www.npr.org/2014/03/06/286378088/reminder-from-a-marine-civilians-and-veterans-share-ownership-of-war.

Kleinman, Arthur, and Robert Desjarlais. 1995. "Violence, Culture, and the Politics of Trauma." In *Writing at the Margin: Discourse Between Anthropology and Medicine*, ed. Arthur Kleinman, 173–89. Berkeley: University of California Press.

Maddow, Rachel. 2012. *Drift: The Unmooring of American Military Power*. New York: Broadway Books.

Mitchell, W. J. T. 1981. *On Narrative*. Chicago: University of Chicago Press.

Mould, Tom. 2012. "Backdoor into Performance." In *The Individual and Tradition: Folkloristic Perspectives*, ed. Ray Cashman, Tom Mould, and Pravina Shukla, 127–43. Bloomington: Indiana University Press.

Noyes, Dorothy. 2011. "Aesthetic Is the Opposite of Anaesthetic: On Tradition and Attention." Paper presented at the Annual Meeting of the American Folklore Society, Bloomington, IN, October 12–15.

Rendon, Jim. 2012. "Post-Traumatic Stress's Surprisingly Positive Flip Side." *New York Times* (March 22). http://www.nytimes.com/2012/03/25/magazine/post-traumatic-stresss-surprisingly-positive-flip-side.html?pagewanted=all.

Shuman, Amy. 2005. *Other People's Stories*. Urbana: University of Illinois Press.

Sontag, Susan. 2003. *Regarding the Pain of Others*. New York: Picador.

Tangherlini, Timothy. 1998. *Talking Trauma*. Jackson: University Press of Mississippi.

Tavernise, Sabrina. 2011. "As Fewer Americans Serve, Growing Gap Is Found Between Civilians and Military." *New York Times* (November 24). http://www.nytimes.com/2011/11/25/us/civilian-military-gap-grows-as-fewer-americans-serve.html?_r=0.

Weiss, Tzipi, and Ron Berger. 2010. *Post-Traumatic Growth and Culturally Competent Practice: Lessons Learned from Around the Globe*. Hoboken, NJ: Wiley.

White, Hayden. 1981. "The Value of Narrativity in the Representation of Reality." In *On Narrative*, ed. W. J. T. Mitchell, 1–25. Chicago, IL: University of Chicago Press.

Young, Katharine. 2006 [1986]. *Taleworlds and Storyrealms*. New York: Springer.

CONTRIBUTORS

Trevor J. Blank is assistant professor of communication at the State University of New York at Potsdam, where he teaches courses in folklore, mass media, and digital culture and researches subversive humor in the vernacular response to traumatic and shocking news events. He is the author of *The Last Laugh: Folk Humor, Celebrity Culture, and Mass-Mediated Disasters in the Digital Age*; coauthor of *Maryland Legends: Folklore from the Old Line State*; editor of the volumes *Folklore and the Internet: Vernacular Expression in a Digital World* and *Folk Culture in the Digital Age: The Emergent Dynamics of Human Interaction*; and coeditor of *Tradition in the Twenty-First Century: Locating the Role of the Past in the Present*. Currently, he serves as editor to the journal *Children's Folklore Review*. Follow him on Twitter @trevorjblank.

Sheila Bock is assistant professor of interdisciplinary studies at University of Nevada, Las Vegas. Her research employs narrative and performance models of analysis to examine how people make sense of their own and others' experiences with health and illness, particularly in contexts of stigma. Specifically, she is interested in how institutional and vernacular framings of such concepts as "culture," "tradition," and "personal experience" work to reify, negotiate, and resist the discursive mechanisms by which certain voices are valued while others, consequently, are dismissed. Her research interests also include foodways, humor, bodylore, and the intersections between folklore and popular culture. Her published work appears in the *Journal of Folklore Research*; *Western Journal of Black Studies*; *Health, Culture, and Society*; the *Journal of Medical Humanities*; the *Journal of Folklore and Education*; and *Western Folklore* (forthcoming 2015).

London Brickley is a doctoral student of folklore and biotechnology at the University of Missouri–Columbia, where she also teaches a variety of culture, film, and literature courses. Her primary research interests and publications focus on the intersections and interplay between folklore, science, and popular culture from the onset of the Enlightenment to the Singularity. She is currently pursuing her inexorably increasing fascination with the biohacking movement by learning, living, and collecting the lore, beliefs, and practices of biopunk's transhuman (r)evolution.

Olivia Caldeira is a PhD candidate in folklore at Memorial University of Newfoundland. She received her MA in comparative studies (with a concentration in folklore) at Ohio State University. Having worked as a direct care provider and a Therapeutic Consultant for young adults with intellectual and developmental disabilities (IDD) experiencing the transition from high school to adulthood, she has witnessed some of the difficulties faced by people with disabilities and their kin and is writing her dissertation based on her fieldwork. She is currently working on two grant committees: one to help job seekers with IDD find meaningful employment and also gather narratives of their successes and struggles, and the other to incorporate Brazilian Jiu Jitsu as one of four recuperative modalities for promoting healing and awareness for people with mind/brain injury and their care networks.

Diane E. Goldstein is professor and chair of the Department of Folklore and Ethnomusicology and director of the Folklore Institute at Indiana University. She is the author of *Once Upon a Virus: AIDS Legends and Vernacular Risk Perception* (2004); coauthor of *Haunting Experiences: Ghosts in Contemporary Folklore* (2008); coeditor of *Reckless Vectors: The Infecting Other in HIV/AIDS Law* (2005); and editor of one of the earliest interdisciplinary HIV/AIDS anthologies, *Talking AIDS: Interdisciplinary Perspectives on Acquired Immune Deficiency Syndrome* (1991). Goldstein's specialties include folk medicine, cultural issues in health care, risk perception, HIV/AIDS, stigmatized illnesses, legend and rumor surrounding health, narrative, ethnography of communications, folklore and violence, folklore and trauma, and applied folklore. She is past president of the American Folklore Society and the International Society for Contemporary Legend Research.

Darcy Holtgrave received her PhD in English with a concentration in folklore from the University of Missouri. Her research interests include digital folklore, personal experience narratives, and mental health advocacy. She serves as the assistant editor for the International Society for Studies in Oral Tradition and SyndicateMizzou at the University of Missouri.

Kate Parker Horigan is assistant professor of folk studies at Western Kentucky University. She was a visiting lecturer in folklore at Indiana University in 2013–2014. She completed her PhD in English with a specialization in folklore at Ohio State University in 2013 and her MA in English at Tulane University in New Orleans in 2006. She is working on a manuscript about the intersections of public trauma, memory, and narrative in post-Katrina New Orleans. Her current research, with support from the Rockefeller Foundation, involves international efforts to improve disaster response by foregrounding the expertise and local knowledge of survivors.

Michael Owen Jones (MA and PhD in folklore) taught courses at UCLA on folk medicine, folk art, food customs, fieldwork, organizational symbolism, and tradition and the individual for forty years until his retirement in 2008. With grants from the National Library of Medicine, he directed a project to digitize Wayland D. Hand's archive of folk medicine, which contains more than two hundred thousand records and is available at www.folkmed.ucla. edu. He also obtained funding from the National Center for Complementary and Alternative Medicine to document Latino folk medicine in Los Angeles. He has authored more than 160 publications. Recent essays concern last meals, aesthetics at home and work, comfort food, and Percy Shelley (the first "celebrity vegan"). Among his books are *People Studying People* (with Robert A. Georges), *Craftsman of the Cumberlands*, *Exploring Folk Art*, *Putting Folklore to Use* (edited), *Folkloristics* (with Robert A. Georges), and *Studying Organizational Symbolism*.

Andrea Kitta is an associate professor at East Carolina University. She is the author of *Vaccinations and Public Concern in History: Legend, Rumor, and Risk Perception*, which won the Brian McConnell Book Award in 2012. Her research on vaccines won the Bernard Duval Prize at the Canadian Immunization Conference. She also participated in the 2012 US–China Exchange Program. She received the Bertie E. Fearing Award for Excellence in Teaching (2010–2011). She is currently working on her next book, *The Kiss of Death: Contamination, Contagion, and Folklore*, to be published by Utah State University Press. Her interests include medical folklore and the folklore of health systems, disability studies, belief, the supernatural, pandemics, stigmatized illnesses, and contemporary legends.

Elaine J. Lawless is Curators' Distinguished Professor and director of the Folklore Program at the University of Missouri. Lawless is an ethnographer who has done field research with religious groups in the American Midwest, the life stories and sermons of clergywomen, and narratives of survivors of domestic violence. Lawless is currently writing her sixth and seventh books, one (with David Todd Lawrence) on Pinhook, Missouri, an African American town that was destroyed in 2011. She is also writing a memoir of her mentor, Professor Winifred Horner, a well-known rhetorician, based on six months of recording Horner's life story until her death in early 2014. In 2003, Lawless created (with Heather Carver, professor of performance studies, University of Missouri) the Troubling Violence Performance Project, a troupe of students who perform actual narratives of domestic violence and sexual assault in order to raise awareness of this taboo subject and encourage dialogue, particularly on college campuses.

Amy Shuman is professor of folklore, English, women's, gender, and sexuality studies and anthropology at Ohio State University, where she also directs the program in disability studies. She is the author of three books: *Storytelling Rights: The Uses of Oral and Written Texts among Urban Adolescents*; *Other People's Stories: Entitlement Claims and the Critique of Empathy*; and *Rejecting Refugees: Political Asylum in the 21st Century* (with Carol Bohmer). Her current projects include a study of the life history narratives told by artisan stonecarvers in Pietrasanta, Italy; research on narratives told by the parents of children with disabilities; and community narrative projects at the intersection of collective memory and public policy.

Annie Tucker is a writer, researcher, and translator investigating the intersections of culture, disability, personal experience, and the arts, primarily in Indonesia. She develops multimodal educational content for Elemental Productions, a documentary film company conducting longitudinal visual psychological ethnography on Java and Bali, and her translation of Indonesian author Eka Kurniawan's novel *Beauty Is a Wound* has been published by New Directions Books. She received her PhD in culture and performance from UCLA's Department of World Arts and Cultures/Dance in 2013 and has been a lecturer for UCLA's growing disability studies minor since 2011.

Kristiana Willsey has a PhD in folklore from Indiana University, where her dissertation focused on issues of entitlement and tellability in veterans' narratives. She is currently a lecturer in the Liberal Arts and Sciences Department of Otis College of Art and Design in Los Angeles, where she teaches courses in children's folklore, fairy tales and new media, and cultural studies. Her research interests also include personal narrative, oral history, oral performance, and poetics.

INDEX

www.ingramcontent.com/pod-product-compliance
Lightning Source LLC
Chambersburg PA
CBHW031127270326
41929CB00011B/1527